Manual of Minor Oral Surgery
A step by step atlas

SCANDINAVIAN UNIVERSITY BOOKS

DENMARK MUNKSGAARD *Copenhagen*

NORWAY UNIVERSITETSFORLAGET *Oslo, Bergen, Tromsø*

SWEDEN ESSELTE STUDIUM *Stockholm, Gothenburg, Lund*

H Birn + J E Winther
Manual of Minor Oral Surgery
A step by step atlas

Munksgaard
Copenhagen

North and South America:
W. B. Saunders Company
Philadelphia / London / Toronto

Manual of Minor Oral Surgery
1. edition, 1. printing 1975

Typesetting: P. J. Schmidt a/s, Vojens
Printing: Villadsen & Christensen, Copenhagen
Cover: Søren Hansen

ISBN 87 16 01805 2

Published simultaneously
in the USA by W. B. Saunders Company

L.C.C.N. 75-18759
ISBN 0-7216-1705-0

Introduction

The objective of this atlas is to give brief guidance in those oral surgery procedures which are considered routine in general practice. It has been written partly for colleagues who are not specialists in oral surgery, and partly for dental students during their clinical training in operation technique. Emphasis has been placed on providing a manual for operation procedures, and problems such as diagnosis, indications and contraindications are mentioned only briefly. For these very important aspects of oral surgery and for more detailed surgical procedures, the reader is kindly referred to comprehensive textbooks on oral surgery.

Manual of Minor Oral Surgery is written on the basis of considerable experience in teaching Scandinavian students according to a Danish book which we published several years ago. The insight gained from using this book in teaching and the helpful criticism we have received along the way have made this English edition possible.

Professor *H. P. Philipsen*, Aarhus, Denmark, has contributed the chapter "Biopsy" and we hereby wish to thank him for his excellent cooperation and for profitable discussions during the preparation of other chapters in this atlas. The constructive criticism and kind editorial advice of professor *M. Shear*, Johannesburg, South Africa, in preparing the English manuscript is greatly appreciated.

Finally we wish to thank the staff of the Department of Oral Surgery for their help and valuable criticism.

Herluf Birn and Jens Erik Winther
Royal Dental College
Aarhus, Denmark
November 1974

Contents

Surgical standard procedures 7
  Incision 7
  Periosteal elevation 11
  Bone resection 11
  Wound debridement 12
  Suture 12
Extraction of teeth 23
Operative removal of roots 34
  The mandible 35
  The maxilla 37
Treatment of abscesses 42
Apicoectomy 47
Cyst operations 53
  Extirpation of cysts 54
  Fenestration of cysts 57
  Removal of mucoceles 63
Exposure of impacted teeth 66
Removal of impacted teeth 73
  The mandibular third molar 74
    The vertical position 76
    The mesio-angular position 79
    The disto-angular position 81
    The horizontal position 84
  The maxillary third molar 86
  The maxillary cuspid 89
  The mandibular cuspid 92
  The second mandibular premolar 94
  The supernumerary tooth 97
Transplantation of teeth 100
Extirpation of labial and lingual frenae 104

Preprosthetic surgery 109
    Alveolar ridge contouring 110
    Intraalveolar resection 114
    Correction of labial and buccal frenae 116
    Removal of fibrous hyperplasia 119
    Removal of denture hyperplasia 120
Closure of sinus perforation 123
Biopsy 126
Index 130

Surgical standard procedures

Certain standard procedures are used in all operations. These will be dealt with in this chapter before the different types of operation are described.

Incision

During the entire incision the scalpel blade must be kept at the desired depth, which most often will mean keeping it in contact with bone. If the cut is repeated several times in the same incision, the wound may easily be lacerated. The incision must be planned with care so that adequate exposure of the operative field can be obtained. Tearing and crushing of the mucosal flap during the operation are thereby avoided. An adequate blood supply must be maintained and the incision should be so planned that the wound may be closed on bony support, even if extensive bone removal is needed.

Furthermore, important structures as the mental nerve, the greater palatine artery and the greater palatine nerve must be localised and avoided during incision.

Fig. 1 In oral surgery a certain number of standard incisions are used, the most simple being the *marginal incision*. This incision is made in the marginal gingiva and is used in areas where the dental arch is concave or straight, i.e. in the entire premolar and molar areas and palatally and lingually in the incisor regions. The scalpel blade is inserted into the gingival crevice and the incision is extended along the buccal or lingual surface of the teeth, thereby cutting the periodontal fibres. The question of whether the interdental papilla should be incised at the base or at the tip merits discussion. As the normal interdental papilla receives adequate blood supply from the underlying bone and periodontal ligament, the incision at the base of the papilla is of no consequence to the survival of tissue. If the incision is carried out in the interdental space, the papilla will invariably be traumatised during elevation of the flap. This may lead to inflammation and formation of negative papillae. As the incision at the base of the papilla is the one which best spares the delicate interdental area, this type should be used in patients with a normal periodontium.

Fig. 2 If however, there is an advanced chronic periodontitis with deep pockets, the blood supply from the bone and periodontal ligament is disturbed and an incision along the tips of the papillae is preferable. This gives better view of the marginal bone and also makes it possible to perform a gingivectomy at the same time, if this should be found necessary. On edentulous alveolar ridges the marginal incision is replaced by an incision along the crest of the alveolar process.

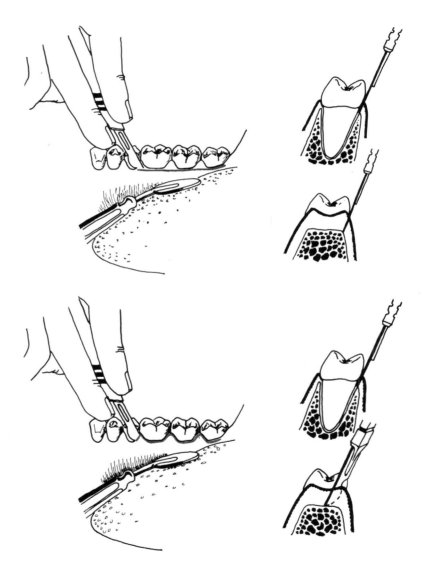

Fig. 3   The *angular incision* is a marginal incision combined with an oblique incision running from the gingival crevice to the buccal or labial sulcus. The oblique incision is placed mesial to the marginal incision so that the operative field is under direct vision. The angular incision is used in flap operations on the facial aspects of the alveolus in both maxilla and mandible. It combines a satisfactory field of vision with adequate blood supply and sufficient stability of the flap during healing. The angle between the marginal and oblique incisions must be obtuse. Note that the oblique incision begins at the base of an interdental papilla in order to ease the placement of suture and lessen the trauma to the marginal gingiva.

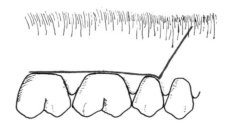

Fig. 4   The *trapezoid incision* is a marginal incision combined with two terminal oblique incisions. It is used in anterior regions of the maxilla and mandible, when large areas of bone have to be exposed, such as in cyst operations and apicoectomies. It is thus used as a substitute for the angular incision in cases where the incision provides inadequate field of vision. The drawing demonstrates the technique. Note again the relationship between the oblique incisions and the interdental papillae. On the right is seen an example of badly planned incisions which result in instability of the mucoperiosteal flap and diminished blood supply.

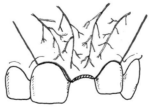 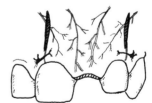

Fig. 5   The *U-formed incision* does not involve the marginal gingiva. It is used in the upper jaw only when there are special indications such as apicoectomies and removal of fractured root tips. The advantage of this incision is that interference with the marginal periodontium is avoided. The incision must be placed at a safe distance from the crevice in order not to jeopardize the blood supply to the gingiva. The accentuated corners of the incision make replacement of flap and suturing easier.

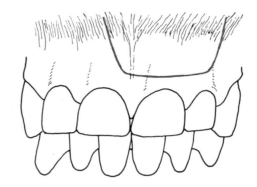

Fig. 6   The *elliptical incision* is used for excision of soft tissue lesions such as tumours and fibrous hyperplasias. It is performed by making two curved incisions which meet at acute angles (see illustration at the right). The incision must be of sufficient length to allow a passive adaptation of the wound edges, even if this necessitates removal of healthy tissue.

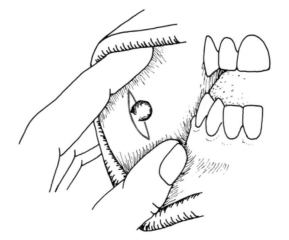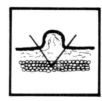

Fig. 7 **Periosteal elevation**

This procedure is used to separate the mucoperiosteal flap from the bone. The periosteal elevator is placed in direct contact with bone through the line of incision. The elevation should start at the gingival margin, primarily loosening all the attached gingiva. The elevation must be atraumatic. If the bone/periosteum attachment is very strong or if the mucosa adheres to underlying pathologic structures, then sharp dissection is indicated.

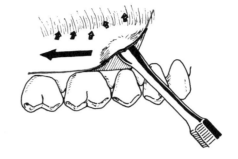

Fig. 8 **Bone resection**

The procedure is carried out using a bur, chisel or *rongeur*. When removing bone with a bur, effective cooling and flushing of the field of operation should be maintained using sterile saline. As an additional safeguard against bone necrosis resulting from overheating, the bur should revolve slowly and be used only intermittently with moderate pressure. Wherever possible a straight handpiece should be used. It offers better vision and less vibration. Note the support from the third and fourth fingers.

The chisel technique requires some training and experience and although there are certain advantages such as minimal heat generation, there are also disadvantages especially of a psychogenic nature for apprehensive patients. The choice between bur and chisel is largely a matter of individual preference based on local custom and training. Chisels must be sharpened each time they have been used. Mallet and chisel are normally used in the mandible only. In the maxilla hand chisels which are more easily controlled are preferred on account of the predominance of cancellous bone. The *rongeur* has a rather limited field of application on account of its size and shape. It is, however, the most atraumatic of all the three types of instruments and should therefore be used as much as possible.

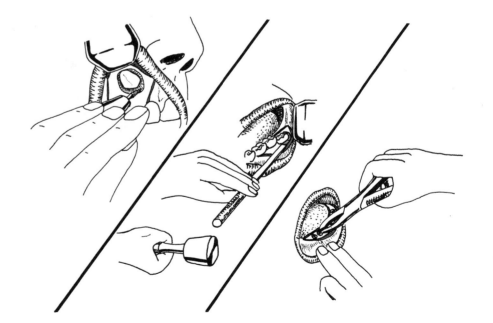

Fig. 9   Wound debridement

Areas of bone which have been traumatized by forceps, elevators or other instruments should have the superficial layer removed as this part of the bone is likely to become necrotic. Sharp crests and spikes which may irritate the overlying mucosa are smoothed and tissue parts with badly disturbed blood supply are removed. Finally, the field of operation is flushed with sterile saline to remove bone chips and foreign bodies which might disturb the healing. It is especially important to irrigate the crevice between the mucoperiosteal flap and the bone.

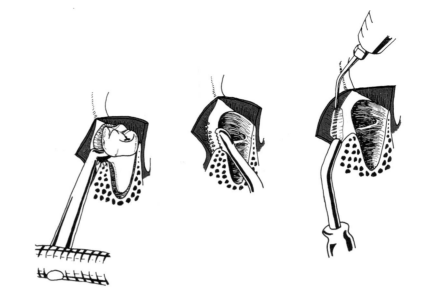

Fig. 10   Suture

In oral surgery, sutures are used mainly for fixation of the wound edges to ensure a primary healing and more seldom to secure hemostasis. It is important that the sutures do not effect a pull in the wound edges, as this could lead to impairment of blood supply with tissue necrosis as a possible result; or the suture material could tear through the mucosa, opening up the wound again. A correct line of incision will in most cases aid in keeping the wound closed with minimal tightening of the sutures. In cases where an absolutely impenetrable cover is needed, as for instance when closing a perforation of the maxillary sinus, it may be necessary to let the sutures exert a gentle pull in the muccsa (see fig. 22 and 23). While a general surgeon uses a wide selection of different suture materials and needles, a dental surgeon working in the oral cavity uses only a few varieties. Silk coated with silicone, and braided polyester are the materials most widely used. One dimension (3–0) of the material preferred and a curved or straight needle complete the instrumentarium. The curved needle is the one most universally used while the straight needle is indicated only for interdental sutures. Catgut may occasionally be used for deep sutures which are completely resorbed. If it is used for mucosal sutures it should be removed like non-resorbable materials, otherwise keloid-

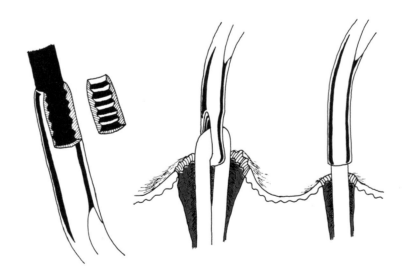

like, hyperplastic tissue may form round the knot. The monofilic nylon has no absorbent effect and therefore creates less inflammation in the surrounding tissue. Owing to its stiffness and smooth surface the nylon suture is, however, difficult to tie and is easily torn through the wound edges. A new type of suture made of polyglycolic acid (Dexon®) has the same advantages as monofilic nylon but it is softer and easier to tie. Furthermore it is resorbable although at a lesser speed than catgut and may be left in places where suture removal is difficult. In certain areas where the mucosa is very thin, the atraumatic suture may be indicated. This is especially true when operating in the floor of the mouth. The atraumatic suture is lead into the needle directly as shown on the drawing. This means that the tissue trauma is less than when a conventional needle with a double suture is pulled through.

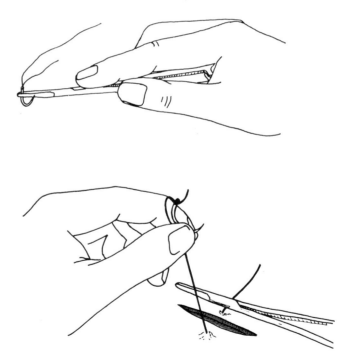

Fig. 11   When suturing has started, the needle is placed in the needle holder as shown on the drawing. In placing the beaks well beneath the eye of the needle there is less risk of fracture in the weak part of the needle.

Fig. 12   The suture most commonly used is the *interrupted suture*. The needle is inserted 3 mm from the wound edge starting in the flap. To avoid tearing the flap the wound edges should be penetrated one at a time. The suture is tied with a surgical knot which, using instrument tie technique, is done in the following way: The suture is drawn through so that the free end is short. The needle holder is placed between the two suture ends.

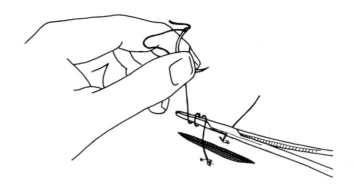

Fig. 13 The long end is twisted twice round the beaks of the needle holder. The coils must be placed peripheral to the lock in order to avoid catching of the suture.

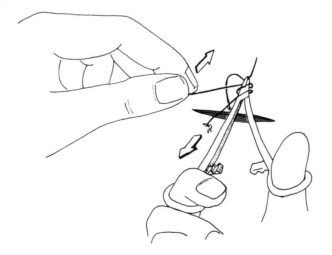

Fig. 14 The short end of the suture is grasped with the needle holder.

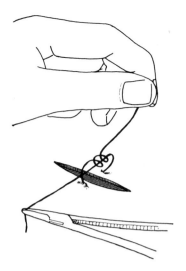

Fig. 15   The needle holder is drawn back through the coils and the two ends of the suture change sides.

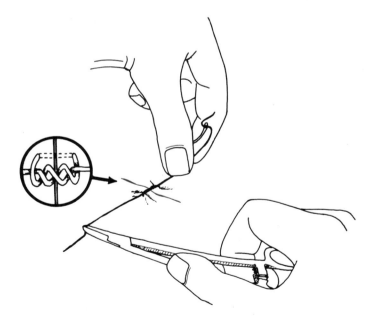

Fig. 16   The knot is tightened and the double twist ensures that it remains that way.

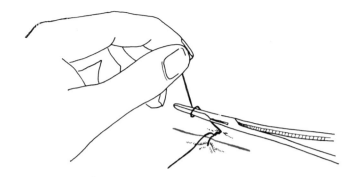

Fig. 17 The needle holder is again placed between the two suture ends and the long one is twisted once round the beaks of the needle holder without pulling on the completed part of the knot.

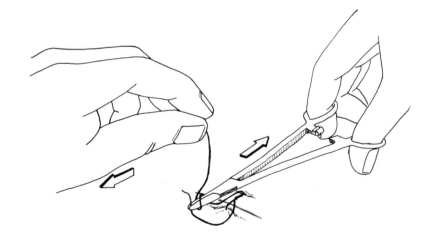

Fig. 18 The short end of the suture is grasped with the needle holder and pulled through the coil.

Fig. 19   The knot is tightened while the two suture ends again change sides. Note that the knot is placed away from the incision. This makes the tightening easier, is less irritating to the wound and facilitates later removal.

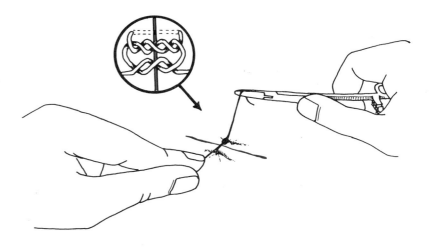

Fig. 20   In order to ease suturing in the attached gingiva it is often an advantage to separate the periosteum from bone in the area of suture placement. This will prevent the needle tearing through the mucosa.

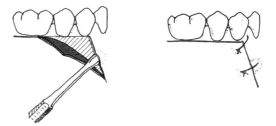

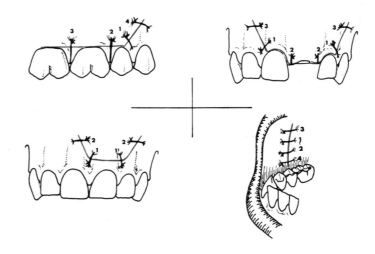

Fig. 21   In order to secure a correct approximation of the wound edges the sutures in the examples shown must be placed in the given order. Note that the corners of the flap are always sutured first. In marginal incisions the order of suturing is unimportant.

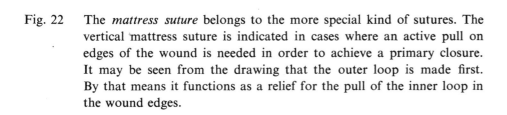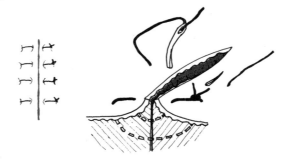

Fig. 22   The *mattress suture* belongs to the more special kind of sutures. The vertical mattress suture is indicated in cases where an active pull on edges of the wound is needed in order to achieve a primary closure. It may be seen from the drawing that the outer loop is made first. By that means it functions as a relief for the pull of the inner loop in the wound edges.

Fig. 23   In cases where closure of soft tissue flaps over bone cavities is needed, such as over extraction sockets or cyst cavities, the horizontal mattress suture is indicated. This suture elevates the wound edges and prevents the mucosal flaps from being inverted into the cavity. At the same time the connective tissue gets a broad contact area and this promotes the healing.

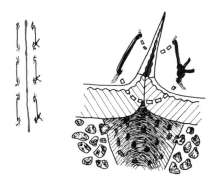

Fig. 24   When closing long incisions the *continuous suture* is often used instead of interrupted sutures. This will produce a neater result in a shorter time. It starts as an interrupted suture, but only the free suture end is cut. The needle end of the suture continues. On the drawing the start of a new loop is illustrated.

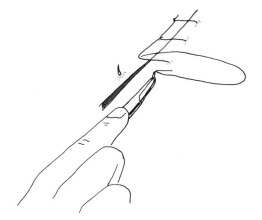

Fig. 25   After cutting through the two wound edges, a loop is formed with fingers of the left hand. The needle holder is passed through the loop to engage the needle.

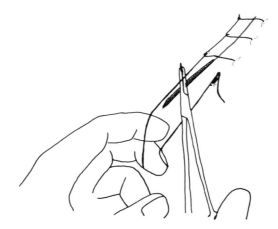

Fig. 26   In order to prevent the loops in the continuous suture slackening after being tightened, the loop may be twisted once before the needle holder is passed through it.

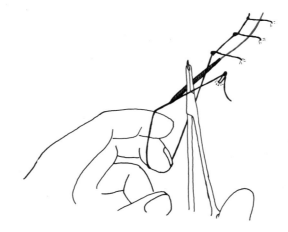

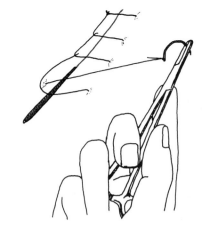

Fig. 27   The needle is pulled back through the loop.

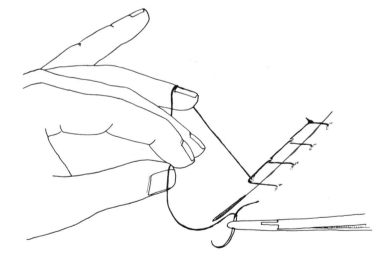

Fig. 28   The suture is tightened so that the loops are placed on the same side of the incision.

Fig. 29   The suture is terminated with a surgical knot as shown on the drawing. Sutures in the oral mucosa can as a rule be removed after 5-7 days.

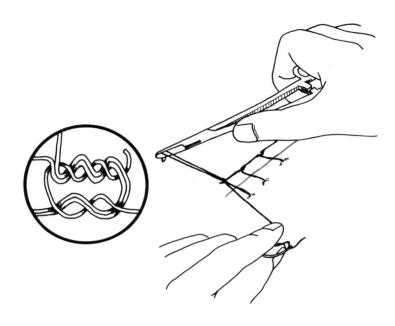

Extraction of teeth

In this chapter a short, systematic outline of the principles involved in extraction of teeth is given. The methods shown may be regarded as standard technique which can be modified according to the experience of the operator and the armamentarium used. A successful extraction implies a thorough knowledge of the dental and alveolar anatomy which may be subject to many variations. A roentgenographic examination is therefore necessary prior to any extraction. – The ultimate goal for any tooth extraction is to break down the dento-alveolar attachment and to overcome the resistance of the bone. To achieve this one must do some movements of luxation with the extraction forceps. We shall distinguish between *rotational movements* and *pendulum movements*, the first ones being rotations of the tooth round the longitudinal axis and the latter being rocking movements in the facio-lingual plane.

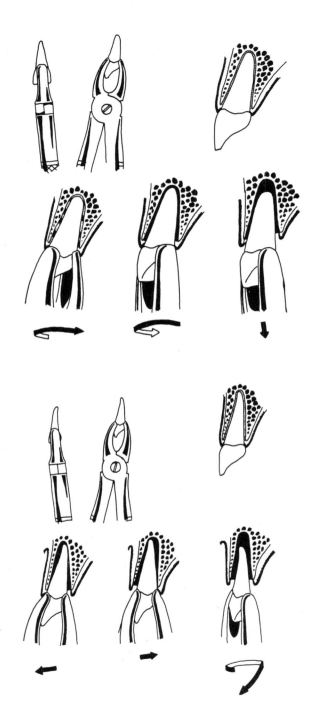

Fig. 30   *The central maxillary incisor* has a conical straight root which in cross section is almost oval. It can be extracted by rotational movements alone. Note in this drawing as in the following that the beaks of the forceps are placed on the root just apical to the cemento-enamel junction.

Fig. 31   *The lateral maxillary incisor* has a slender root which is oval in cross section. There is often a distal curvature of the root tip. It may be extracted by pendulum movements which in the terminal stage can be substituted by slight rotation in mesial direction turning the tooth out of the alveolus.

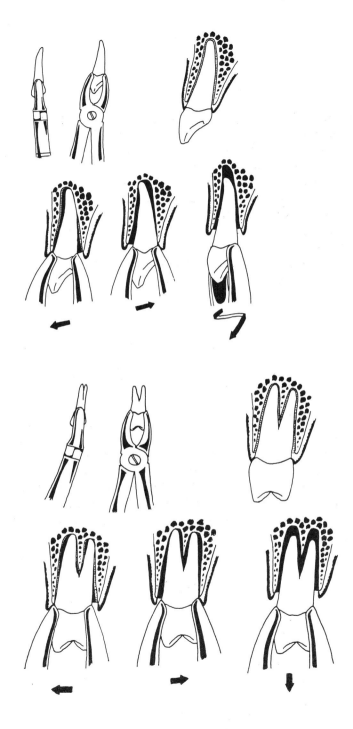

Fig. 32   *The maxillary cuspid* has a long, sturdy root which is triangular in cross section and often with a disto-labial curvature of the root tip. The labial alveolar wall of compact bone is very thin especially in the marginal area, and there is a considerable risk of fracturing the bone during luxation. If the tooth is very firmly anchored in the socket, it is advisable to do a flap operation and remove part of the labial bone before continuing the extraction. The tooth is extracted using pendulum movements terminated by careful rotation depending on the degree of root tip curvature.

Fig. 33   *The first maxillary premolar* often has a bifid root with slender root tips. It should be handled with caution using pendulum movements only and any attempt at rotation is contraindicated.

Fig. 34   If the root tips of the first maxillary premolar are fractured they can often be removed like other root tips with a slender root-tip pick. The removal is easier if the root tips are slightly loosened before the fracture. This is one of the reasons for caution during the first part of the extraction. The point of the pick is wedged into the periodontal space using the most coronally placed part of the fracture as a starting point. The root is loosened with small movements of the elevator and drawn out of the socket as shown to the right. Neither the elevator nor the surrounding bone can withstand great pressure, and if the root tips are not loosened within a resonable time they should be removed by labial flap operation.

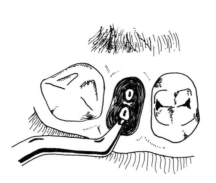
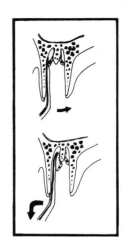

Fig. 35   *The second maxillary premolar* has a short conical root which is oval in cross section. The extraction is started by pendulum movements, but because of the often close relationship between the root tip and the maxillary sinus, it is continued by rotational movements which are less likely to create a communication between the socket and the antrum.

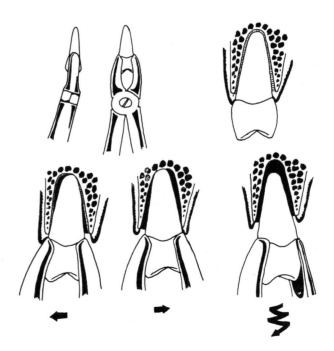

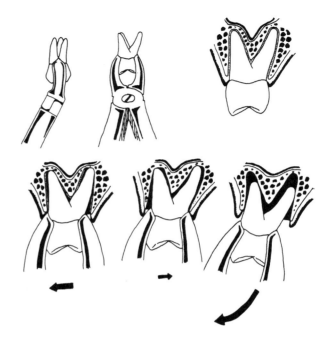

Fig. 36   Extraction of the *first and the second maxillary molars* is described under one heading as the differences in anatomy of roots and alveolar bone do not warrant any principal differences in method of extraction. Of the three roots, the palatal is the most sturdy and often diverges considerably from the two buccal roots. The buccal bone is rather thin except at the infrazygomatic crest. The surrounding bone is cancellous and easily compressed. The root tips have as a rule a very close relationship to the maxillary sinus, and it is in this region that sinus perforations most often occur. The extraction is carried out by applying pendulum movements, predominantly in a buccal direction where the resistance is the least. The tooth is removed from the socket connection with a buccally directed turn following the curvature of the palatal root.

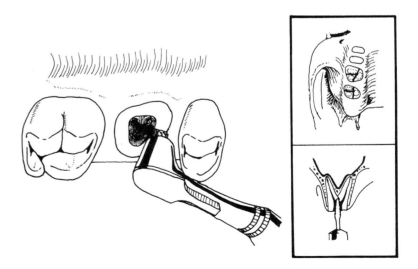

Fig. 37   If the molar is very firmly anchored in the socket, or if the crown is so destroyed by caries that an adequate grip of the forceps is impossible, it is necessary to divide the tooth and remove the roots one by one. The success of this procedure is dependent upon the roots being clearly separated and their having uncomplicated anatomical configurations. The division is started in the subpulpal wall, from where the bur is led towards the periphery mesially and distally. Note the difference in the size of the mesio-buccal roots on the first and the second molar which influence the line of division. After cutting off the palatal root, the buccal roots are separated. In view of the close relation to the maxillary sinus the bur should not penetrate the subpulpal wall. The last bridge of dentine can be fractured by a slight rotation of the elevator in the crevice.

Fig. 38   The disto-buccal root is removed by tilting the elevator using the palatal root as support. The mesio-buccal root is best removed by placing the elevator mesially and directing the root into a distally aimed curvature. This is made possible by the space created after removal of the disto-buccal root. It is important that the force is directed so that the root is dislodged in an outward direction as when the anatomical conditions are unfavourable only a little pressure is needed to press the root into the maxillary sinus. If the preoperative radiograph reveals that only a thin bony partition exists, the roots should be removed by flap operation and resection of a part of the buccal bone.

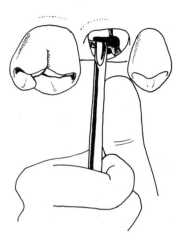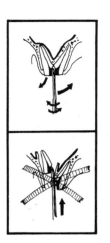

Fig. 39   The palatal root can usually be rotated out of the socket using a root forceps with slender beaks. This procedure is less risky than using an elevator, which may displace the root into the sinus.

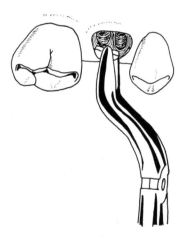

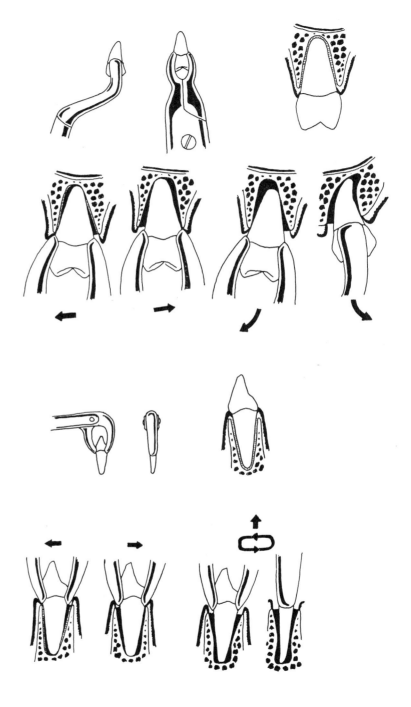

Fig. 40 *The third maxillary molar* is situated in the highly cancellous bone of the tuberosity, and its root anatomy is subject to wide variations. If three or more roots are present, it may be extracted in the way described for the two other molars, but very often it has only one conical root with a distally directed curvature which necessitates a distal turn during removal. If a sinus perforation is suspected after extraction of maxillary molars, proper diagnostic measures should be applied to confirm or disconfirm this. If a perforation is found, it is treated according to the directions given on page 123.

Fig. 41 *The mandibular incisors* have a delicate root which is flat in mesio-distal direction and is surrounded by thin lamellar bone labially and lingually. These conditions indicate a very cautious extraction to avoid fracture of bone or root. The luxation is done by small pendulum movements which are replaced – when some mobility has been achieved – by ellipsoid motions as indicated on the drawing. These motions are used to enlarge the marginal bone in the alveolus.

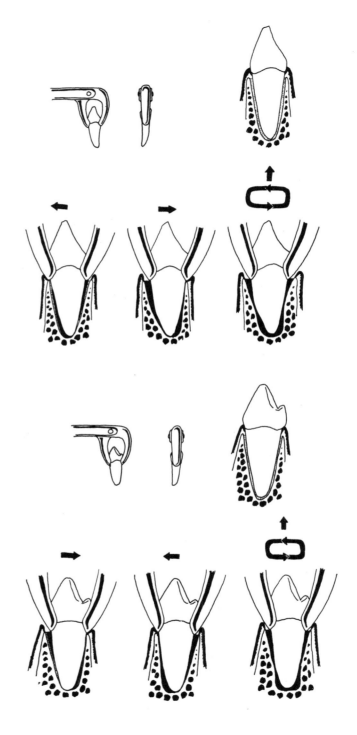

Fig. 42   *The mandibular cuspid* has a sturdy taproot and is, like the incisors, surrounded by thin lamellar bone. The principles of extraction are therefore similar to those governing the extraction of incisors, i.e. introductory small pendulum movements terminated by ellipsoid motions.

Fig. 43   *The first mandibular premolar* has a sturdy root which is oval in cross section. The buccal lamellar bone is now gaining in thickness. The incongruity between the curvature of the mandibular dental arch and the mandibular body and the presence of the oblique line leads to an increase in thickness and strength of the buccal alveolar bone when moving distally in the dental arch. The resistance to extraction will lie in the marginal part of the alveolus as the amount of cancellous bone in the apical region is rather liberal. The first mandibular premolar is extracted using pendulum movements followed by ellipsoid or rotary motions to remove the tooth from its socket.

Fig. 44　*The second mandibular premolar* has a conical relatively short root which is almost circular in cross section. This tooth may therefore be rotated out of its socket after very few pendulum movements. The marginal ring of lamellar bone is accordingly of little importance.

Fig. 45　*The mandibular molars* have sturdy roots flattened in mesiodistal direction. They may have a slight distal curvature and can be extracted after identical principles. The teeth are firmly anchored especially because of the thickness of the buccal alveolar bone. It is necessary to put power behind the pendulum movements which are directed predominantly to the lingual side. The actual removal of the tooth from its socket is best achieved in a buccal direction.

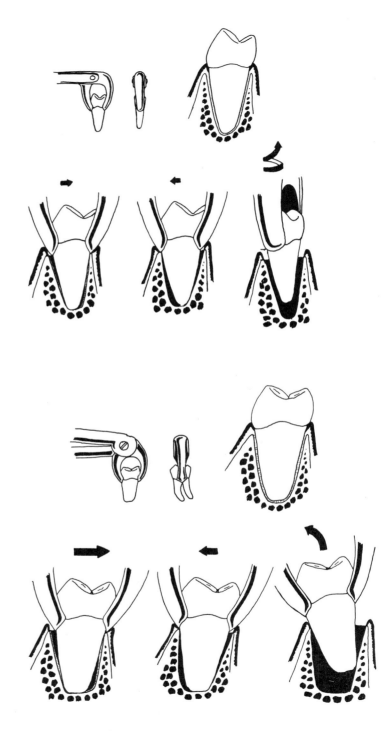

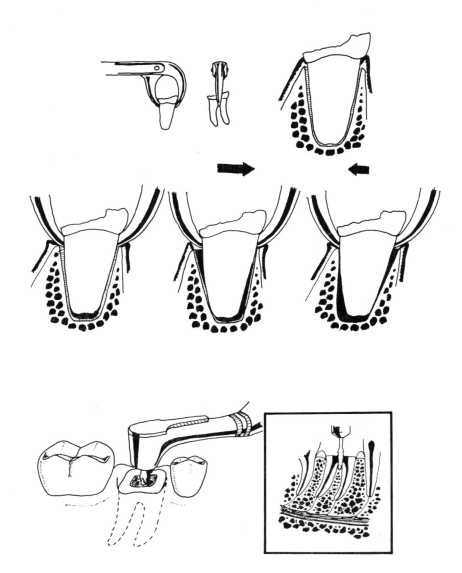

Fig. 46 Heavily destroyed mandibular molars are best extracted with a *cow-horn forceps*, where the beaks are pressed down into the bifurcation. This gives a better grip on the tooth than when using an ordinary forceps. The extraction motions are however the same as described earlier (Fig. 45). If the tooth is very weak in the bifurcation the cowhorn forceps may separate the two roots from each other. Removal of the tooth may then be undertaken according to the guidelines in the following figures (Fig. 48 and 49).

Fig. 47 When an extraction with forceps has to be abandoned, division of the tooth, followed by removal of the roots one by one, is the treatment of choice. Using a bur, the roots are separated by a deep crevice which extends into the interradicular septum. The cut starts in the subpulpal wall and the bur is drawn towards the periphery.

Fig. 48   Barry's elevator is placed deep in the crevice. The distal root is removed first because it normally yields the lesser resistance of the two and also has the most favourable root curvature in relation to the path of removal. Note that the support of the elevator lies on the mesial root.

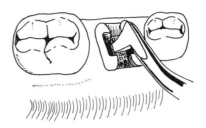 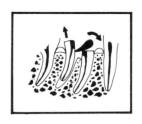

Fig. 49   The mesial root can now be removed by placing Barry's elevator in the empty socket and perforating the interdental septum if necessary with the tip of the elevator. By cautions rotation of the elevator handle the root is pushed upwards. The interdental septum is inspected and potentially loose pieces of bone are removed. If the bony septum is grossly damaged it should be removed using a *rongeur*.

Finally it may be emphasized once more that the principles of extraction described here must be regarded as directional only as many unforeseen anatomical and physical factors may necessitate individual changes in procedure. The fine nuances of extraction technique must in each case always be directed by the particular kind of resistance encountered during the initial motions. The movements of the tooth are increased in the direction of least resistance, so that one tries to find the most expeditious method of extraction. If multiple extractions are planned, it is advantageous to remove the maxillary teeth prior to the mandibular teeth and to start distally in the dental arch.

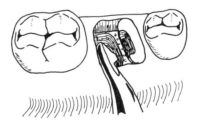 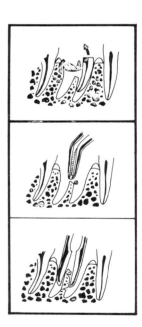

Operative removal of roots

In many cases an operative removal will prove less traumatizing than continued unsuccessful attempts at intraalveolar extraction. The wound healing will, when a correct operation technique is used, proceed faster and result in a smoother remodelling of the alveolar process. The method of operation is essentially the same, whether it concerns uni- or multirooted teeth. However, in view of differences between the maxilla and mandible in bone structure and relations to other anatomical structures, the technique will be different in the two jaws.

The operation consists of the following phases:

1) Reflection of mucoperiosteal flap
2) Denudation of a suitable part of the root
3) Extraction with elevator or root forceps
4) Wound debridement and suture

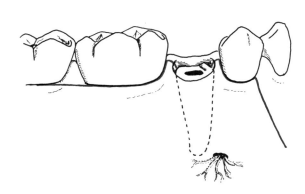

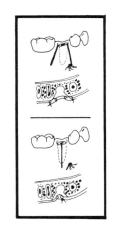

Fig. 50 **The mandible**

Angular incisions are usually used. Note how the incision avoids the region of the mental foramen, which may be situated in various places from under the mesial root tip of the first molar to under the root tip of the first premolar. To the right are seen two examples of improper incisions which both yield an unsatisfactory view of the field of operation and also cause unsupported wound edges.

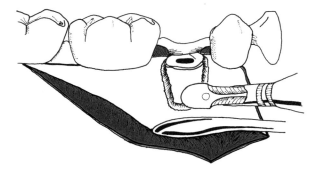

Fig. 51 The mucoperiosteal flap is reflected and the buccal bone is removed with a bur to expose approximately one half of the root. Note the placement of the periosteal elevator to protect the soft tissue and the mental nerve.

Fig. 52 The buccal bone has been removed and the full mesio-distal width of the root exposed. To facilitate the use of elevators a hole is made into the root at the apical end of the bony window. Note the inclined direction of the cut which gives the most efficient utilization of the force of the elevator.

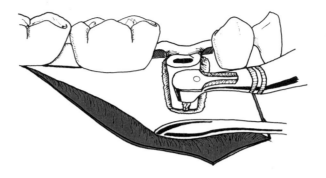

Fig. 53 With a contra-angled elevator placed in the cut and the buccal bone shelf as support, the root can now be elevated. If the root tip is curved in a distal or mesial direction it may often be necessary to apply the elevator on the mesial or distal side of the root respectively.

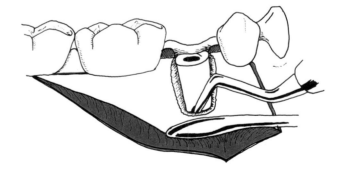

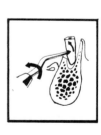

Fig. 54   After wound debridement the sutures are placed as shown on the drawing. Note the position of the interdental sutures with firm bone support and not across the opening of the alveolus. The suture in the vertical incision must draw upwards to the marginal gingiva, so that the wound edges are placed in correct relation to each other.

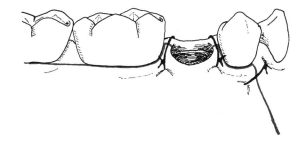

Fig. 55   **The maxilla**
The angular incision is also used most frequently here, although the trapezoid incision may be indicated in the anterior region.

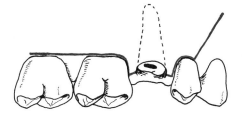

Fig. 56   The root is exposed in the manner previously mentioned. A hand piece is used here and should be preferred wherever adequate space is available. Close relationship between the root tip and the maxillary sinus is no contraindication to this technique, but rather adds to the indication for operation to ensure atraumatic removal.

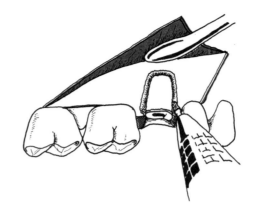

Fig. 57   The root may be removed with a straight elevator which is wedged into the periodontal space on the palatal side, where the bone is of adequate strength to withstand the pressure. Luxation of the root is accomplished by rotating the elevator using very little pressure in the apical direction.

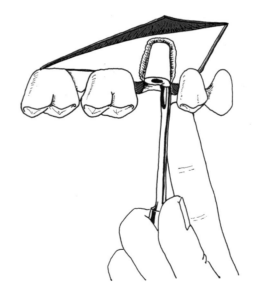
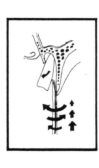

Fig. 58 The root may also be removed with a root forceps which is placed as shown on the figure. This grip combined with an adequate bone removal ensures that the root can be extracted in the most favourable direction with only a limited application of force.

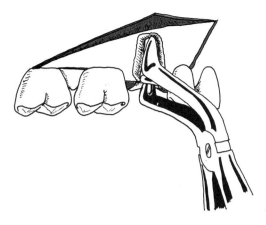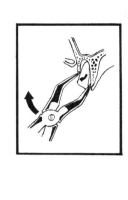

Fig. 59 The sutures are placed according to the guidelines previously described for the mandible. A supplementary suture in the unattached mucosa may be necessary if the vertical incision has been extended more than usual, or if the wound edges do not adapt closely do each other.

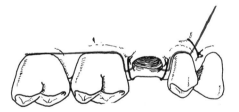

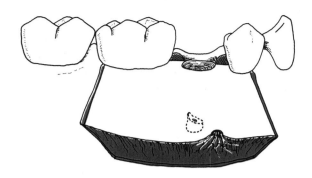

Fig. 60   In cases where only the apical fragment is left in the socket, the technique may be modified in some ways. As one example a hypercementotic root tip from a mandibular premolar is shown. The trapezoid incision is indicated here as it yields a larger bone exposure and thereby a better view into the operative area.

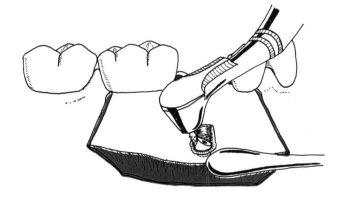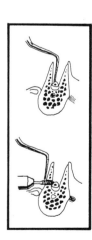

Fig. 61   It is now possible to expose the root tip through a bony window avoiding loss of marginal bone. The exact location of the root tip may be found using a periodontal probe as shown on the right side of the drawing.

Fig. 62   The root tip is exposed almost completely and removed with a contra-angled root pick through the buccal window. To ensure adequate closure at least two sutures are necessary in the vertical incisions.

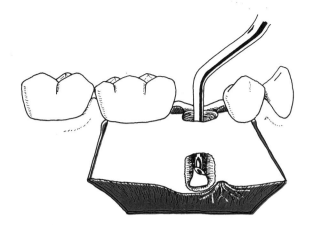

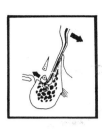

Treatment of abscesses

The only effective treatment of abscesses is still surgical incision and drainage in spite of the influence that modern chemotherapy has had on the treatment of infections. The microorganisms in an abscess are not readily accessible for antibiotics and a treatment with these compounds may only give a false security and cloud the true character of the infection. In certain cases chemotherapy may be indicated to support the surgical treatment. As a method for pain control during the incision, regional local analgesia is preferred whenever it is possible to bypass the abscess with a needle. The local analgesia may be supplemented or even replaced by general analgesia with nitrous oxide, whereas any method of topical analgesia is worthless. It is not the covering mucosa as much as the very sensitive base of the abscess which elicits the pain.

The treatment consists of the following phases:
1) Incision
2) Exploration and pus discharge
3) Drainage

Fig. 63　With a lancet or a straight pointed scalpel the incision is done in the most dependant area to ensure an optimal drainage later on. The incision should be made from the side towards the centre to avoid too much pressure on the sensitive base. The knife must not be carried too deep into the abscess and enlargement of the incision can be done during withdrawal to avoid destroying deeper structures.

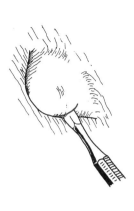
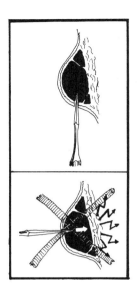

Fig. 64　In order to achieve an effective discharge of pus from all parts of the abscess a Lister forceps is introduced into the incision. During probing in the cavity, pockets of pus are drained by opening the beaks of the forceps.

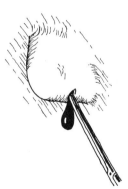
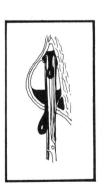

Fig. 65   To secure a continued drainage from the cavity a piece of rubber dam is introduced through the incision. The drain should only fill out part of the cavity space. It must be kept in place with a suture to avoid it being dislodged from the cavity. The drain should be kept in place for two days after which the acute infection has usually subsided to such an extent that the cause of the infection can be treated.

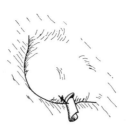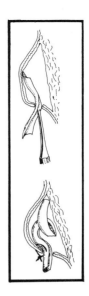

Fig. 66   The dental abscess often presents itself in the labial and buccal vestibule. Normally there are no important structures to take into consideration and the incision may therefore be placed according to the demand for the best possible drainage. As shown on the drawing the scalpel is introduced into the abscess parallel to the alveolar process. In the premolar and molar region of the mandible care should be exercised to avoid damage to the mental nerve and the facial artery and vein.

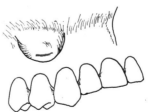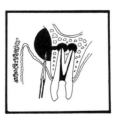

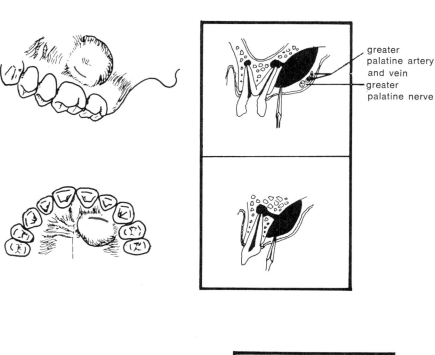

greater palatine artery and vein
greater palatine nerve

Fig. 67   Incision of palatal abscesses demands special consideration towards the greater palatine vein, artery and nerve. These structures are located superficial to the abscess which will form between the bone and the periosteum. The incision is therefore placed near the marginal gingiva parallel to the dental arch.

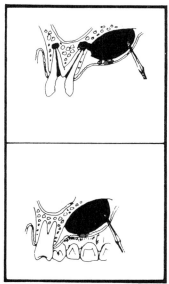

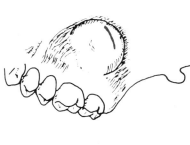

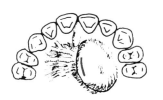

Fig. 68   In cases where the abscess is situated at some distance from the marginal gingiva closer to the midline the incision should be placed medially parallel to and close to the midline.

Fig. 69   Abscesses in the sublingual region are most frequently found in the premolar and first molar regions. Among the important structures in this area should be mentioned the sublingual gland, the submandibular duct and the sublingual artery. To avoid damage to these structures the incision is placed parallel to the dental arch as shown in the drawing, and the requirement for optimal drainage in this region has therefore to be disregarded. Note the inclined direction of the scalpel as a further security measure against damage to the structures in the floor of the mouth.

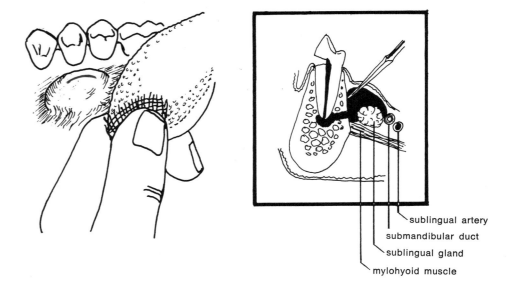

sublingual artery
submandibular duct
sublingual gland
mylohyoid muscle

Apicoectomy

Apicoectomy is only regarded as a supplement to normal endodontic therapy and can therefore never replace it.

The treatment consists of the following phases:

1) Reflection of a muco-periosteal flap
2) Exposure of the periapical region of the tooth involved
3) Curettage of pathologic tissue
4) Resection of the apical part of the root tip
5) Closure of the root canal
6) Wound debridement, suture and control radiographs
7) Patient follow-up

Fig. 70   In the anterior part of the maxilla where most apicoectomies are performed, a U-shaped incision is preferred. To ensure proper healing the incision must be placed well outside the expected border of the bone cavity so that sutures may be placed on solid bone. Consideration of the marginal gingiva dictates also that there is an adequate strip of attached gingiva left outside the flap. If these demands cannot be met either because of the size of the bony defect or as a result of marginal bone loss, a trapezoid incision is preferred as shown to the right of the figure. If periodontal surgery is indicated this should be carried out as part of the operation.

In the posterior region of the mandible an angular incision is preferred while in the anterior region a trapezoid incision is appropriate.

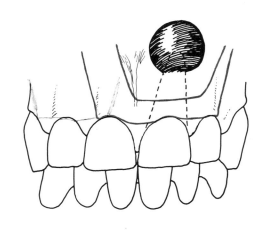
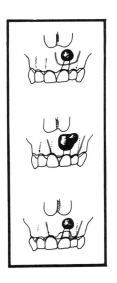

Fig. 71   The flap reflection is carried out as described earlier, but if the pathologic process has penetrated the bone and as such is adherent to the periosteum, the mucosal flap must be disengaged by blunt dissection. If fistulous tracts are present they should be cut close to the bone. Excision of the tract in the mucosa is contraindicated. This will only create a larger perforation which disturbs the healing. The fistula will close gradually after the cause has been removed.

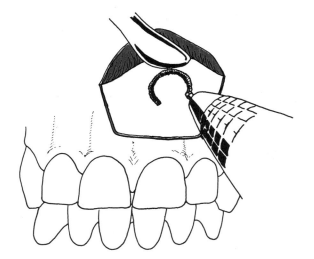

Fig. 72   If the labial cortical plate is intact the root tip may be localized by the rule of thumb that the root length is 1½ times the crown length. For orientation in the mesio-distal direction the alveolar juga may be used. The penetration of the bone is normally done with a bur, but if the overlying bone cover is thin and the pathological process of a reasonably large dimension such as is sometimes seen in cysts, a bone *rongeur* can be used very atraumatically and efficiently.

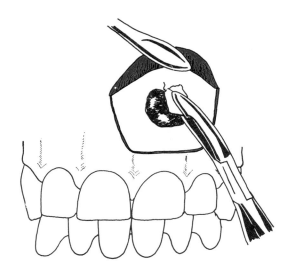

Fig. 73   Removal of bone is carried out to an extent which gives an easy access to the whole of the pathological process. Granulomatous tissue can now be removed with a curette.

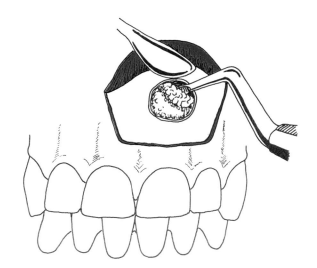

Fig. 74   If a cyst is present a periosteal elevator or large curette is placed between the lining of the cyst and the bone and the whole sac is gently disengaged from the cavity walls and lifted out. To avoid perforation of the cyst, the curette is placed with the convex side towards the lining in the initial stages of the enucleation.

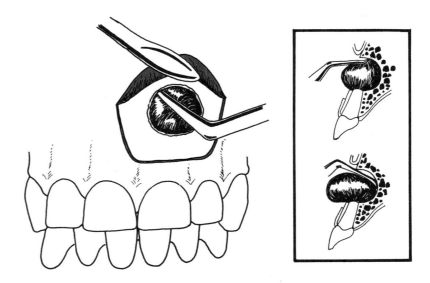

Fig. 75   Part of the root tip including the apical ramifications of the root canal is cut off with a bur. It is not necessary to resect all of the root exposed in the pathological cavity. The cut is made with a labial inclination which gives an adequate view of the apical foramen.

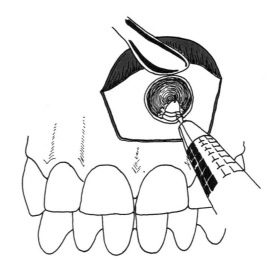

Fig. 76   On completing the resection, the remnants of pathological tissue which until now have been difficult to approach are removed. A Kaplan periodontal instrument may prove useful here. The root canal is now cleaned with reamers and files whether or not there is an existing root filling. The canal is irrigated and dried with alcohol. Before a new root filling is placed, the apical area should be packed with hemostatic gauze to minimize the bleeding. A guttapercha point is pushed through the apical foramen to seal it off completely. The root filling is completed in the usual manner and finally the excess of guttapercha point is cut off with a hot instrument.

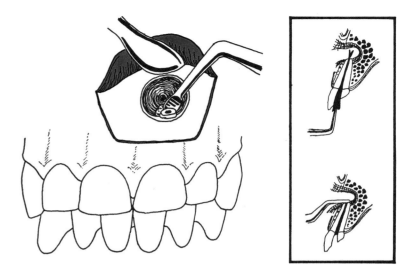

Fig. 77   If the root canal is obliterated for one or another reason, the apical part of the canal is closed with a retrograde silver amalgam root filling. A non zinc type of amalgam is preferred owing to the difficulties in keeping the field completely sealed off. With a miniature contra-angle handpiece, a cavity with undercut walls is prepared in the root canal. The cavity should be at least 2 mm deep following the long axis of the root. The cut root surface may be smoothened prior to insertion of the amalgam filling using a vulcanite bur operating at great speed. This will give a well defined borderline for the filling. The operative area is packed with hemostatic gauze and the root canal is filled. The filling is carved and all excessive amalgam carefully removed.

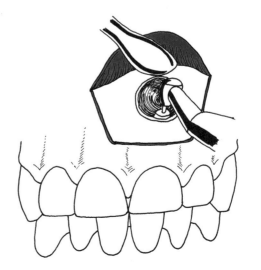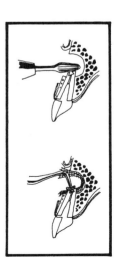

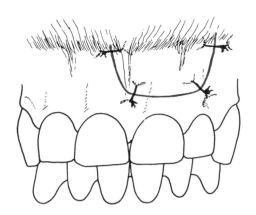
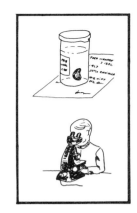

Fig. 78   The sutures are placed as shown on the drawing. The pathological tissue should be sent for microscopic examination.

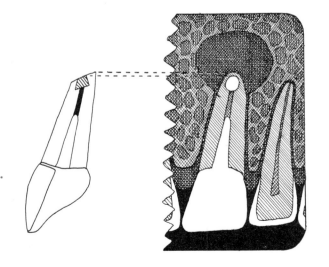

Fig. 79   The healing of the periapical area is evaluated by yearly radiographic examinations until bone has filled in satisfactorily. In order to evaluate the progress a postoperative radiograph is essential. As a result of the inclination of the resected apical surface the radiograph may show a root filling which apparently does not reach the apex. The explanation of this phenomenon is seen from the figure.

Cyst operations

There are two different principles involved in the treatment of cysts: extirpation and fenestration (marsupialization). Extirpation of a cyst consists of the total removal of the cyst lining and a primary closure of the bone cavity. In fenestration of a cyst a permanent connection between the cyst and the oral cavity is created and maintained by means of an obturator. The expansive growth of the cyst is thereby stopped and a gradual reduction of the cystic cavity takes place concurrently with regeneration of bone. The cyst epithelium, which for the most part is left untouched, is gradually transformed to an oral epithelium.

Fig. 80 **Extirpation of cysts**

Extirpation is used in cases where the operation may be carried out without damage to the neighbouring structures and it is therefore not only the size of the cyst as such which is decisive in determining the method of operation.

The operation consists of the following phases:

1) Reflection of muco-periosteal flap
2) Exposure of part of the cyst
3) Enucleation of the cyst
4) Inspection of the cyst lining and cavity
5) Wound debridement and suture
6) Annual follow-up of healing

To illustrate this method of operation we have chosen a radicular cyst from a grossly carious maxillary right lateral incisor which is to be extracted. Cyst extirpation in connection with apicoectomy has been described previously (Fig. 70–79).

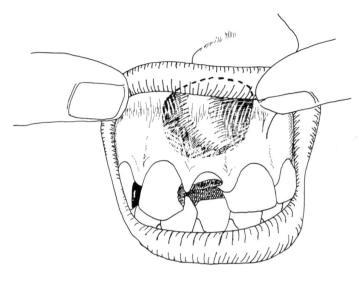

Fig. 81   After extraction of the tooth a trapezoid incision is made. Note that the interdental papillae are cut at their crests (see Fig. 2).

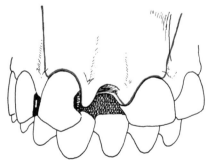

Fig. 82   The muco-periosteal flap is reflected. If the cyst lining is adherent to the submucosal layer a blunt dissection is carried out with scissors. The closed instrument is placed between the periosteum and the cyst. The scissors are then opened and withdrawn and the two structures are thereby separated.

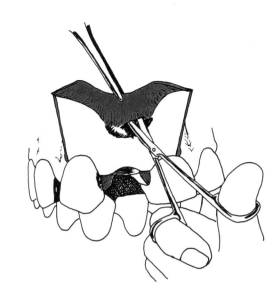

Fig. 83   The opening in the bone is enlarged using a *rongeur* which best protects the membrane against damage. Bone is removed to such extent that there is easy access to all parts of the cyst cavity. If the bone cover is intact, the primary opening is made with a bur as shown in Fig. 71.

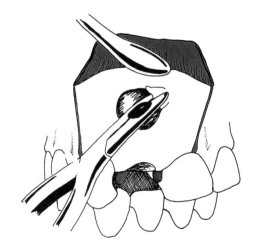

Fig. 84 For extirpation of small cysts a curette may be used while larger cysts are better enucleated with a periosteal elevator as shown on the drawing. Any possible adherence to the palatal mucosa is disengaged with a pair of scissors.

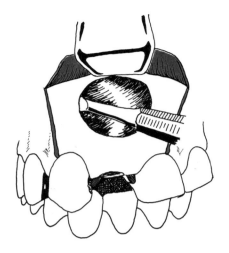
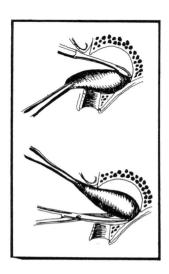

Fig. 85 Following the extirpation the cavity is inspected and irrigated with saline. The sutures are placed as shown. Note that the alveolus is left open. The cyst lining is sent for histological examination. Radiologic follow-up of the healing is carried out at yearly intervals.

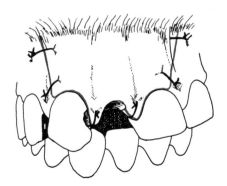

Fig. 86 **Fenestration of cysts**

Fenestration is used when it may be assumed that extirpation would damage important neighbouring structures such as apices of vital teeth, the maxillary sinus and the inferior alveolar nerve. Another important indication for fenestration is the treatment of dentigerous cysts in cases where the tooth involved should be preserved and helped to erupt.
The operation consists of the following phases:
1) Cutting out a window in the cyst wall
2) Construction and insertion of an obturator
3) Patient follow-up
As an example we have chosen a radicular cyst from the lateral incisor with very close relations to the apices of the neighbouring teeth.

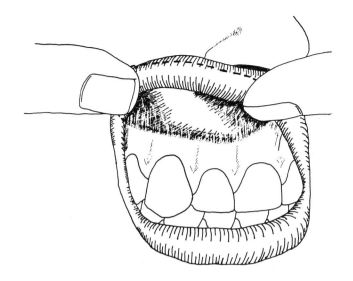

Fig. 87 In such cases where the causative tooth is to be preserved, the actual treatment of the cyst must be preceded by an apicoectomy with a conventional or retrograde root filling. The drawing shows the line of incision. The dimension of the trapezoid incision depends on the extent to which the cyst has penetrated the cortical plate. This may be diagnosed by palpation. The line of incision shown here is the least permissible.

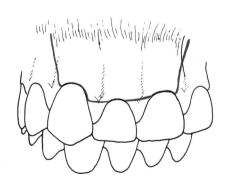

Fig. 88 The cyst is exposed to an extent involving the periapical area of the tooth and the site for the obturator to come. The exposed part of the cyst lining is excised and sent for histological examination.

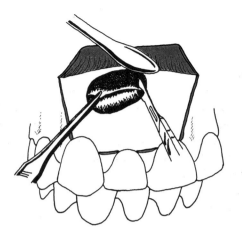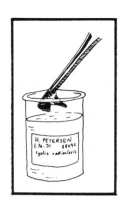

Fig. 89 The remaining part of the cyst wall is inspected thoroughly for hyperplastic areas or other suspicious alterations. If these are present they should be excised and sent for histological examination. The root-tip is amputated, and the root canal filled according to the guidelines previously mentioned (Fig. 75–77).

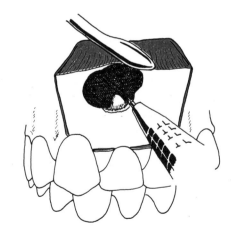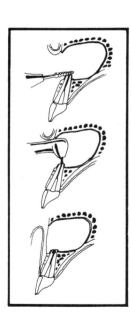

Fig. 90   The muco-periosteal flap is secured with sutures as shown on the drawing. A window is now cut out which has the same dimension as the obturator. The opening must be placed near the labial fold at an adequate distance from the roots of the teeth. A close relationship between the obturator and a root surface may expose the cementum and leave a denuded area which will later be exposed to carious destruction. The best position is normally between the roots as shown on the drawing.

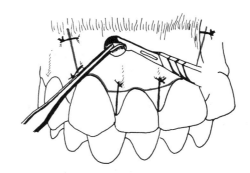

Fig. 91   The obturator is made and inserted immediately after the operation. Using premanufactured acrylic tubes, the usual procedure of taking an impression and having an intermediate period with gauze pack may be avoided. The tube is pushed through the opening and made to fit the depth of the cavity with adequate space to the distal wall.
In one end of the tube retention holes are drilled and selfpolymerizing acrylic is used to form a collar round the tube.

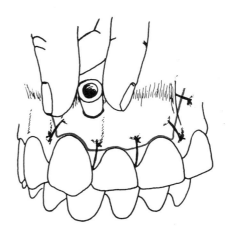
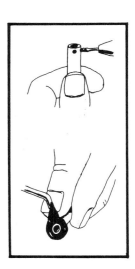

Fig. 92   While the acrylic is still soft the other end of the tube is inserted and the collar contoured to the structures surrounding the opening, especially in the labial fold. After the acrylic has set, the plate is polished and the obturator is completed. The patient may now take out the obturator without discomfort, flush the cavity with lukewarm, boiled water and reinsert it. This should be done twice a day. After initial postoperative examination for decubital ulcers, healing of the cyst cavity should be followed at 1–2 month intervals. In children and adolescents the bone regeneration is fast and therefore frequent visits are necessary. The obturator is shortened as the size of the cyst cavity is reduced. The final result may be a depression in the oral mucosa following the discontinuation of the obturator treatment. There is, however, more likely to be a tubelike remnant of the cavity which requires a surgical correction for hygienic reasons.

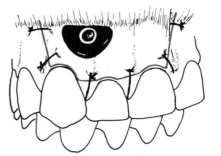
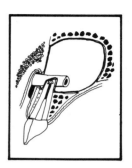

Fig. 93   If a cyst in an edentulous jaw requires fenestration, the obturator may be fastened to the denture. As an example we have chosen a residual cyst in the mandible in close relation to the neurovascular bundle.

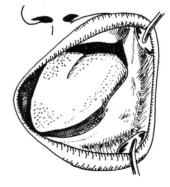
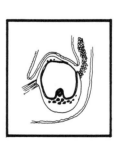

Fig. 94   One of the prosthetic teeth immediately above the cyst is removed and the hole is carried through the denture base. The denture is inserted and the position of the future obturator is marked on the mucosa. The opening to the cyst cavity is now made with a pointed scalpel which is capable of penetrating thin layers of bone, too. If the bone cover is thick a bur may be used .The excised tissue including part of the cyst lining is now submitted for histological examination.

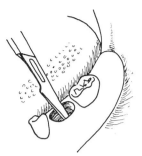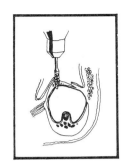

Fig. 95   To avoid food impaction into the cyst cavity an acrylic stick of the same dimension as the formerly described tube is used. This stick is fitted and attached to the denture with selfpolymerizing acrylic. After setting the acrylic is polished and the obturator is completed. It is important that the direction of the stick is parallel to the line of insertion of the denture. A part of the obturator may sometimes be left as extra retention. In these cases, however, a relining should be made to ensure an optimal fit. The acrylic tubes or sticks are available from manufacturers of plastic materials and may be sterilized in the autoclave.

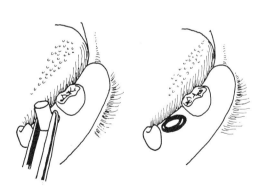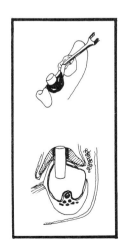

Fig. 96   Fenestration of cysts is, at least in adult patients, a very slow treatment which may last from 2–4 years. In view of this inconvenience to the patient and with regard to the problems discussed in Fig. 92 a secondary operation is often indicated at an earlier stage, when bone regeneration has covered the structures which were the concern at the first operation. The present figure shows a residual cavity after fenestration of the cyst described in Figs. 86–92. A U-formed incision is made at an adequate distance from the cavity.

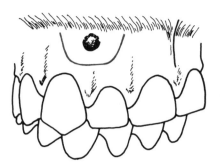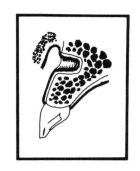

Fig. 97   The muco-periosteal flap is reflected together with the mucosal lining in the tubelike cavity. The last remnants of epithelial tissue in the bottom of the cavity are now removed. The mucosal lining of the tubelike cavity which is now part of the mucoperiosteal flap is turned inside out or evaginated, resulting in a broad area of contact between the connective tissue in the tube.

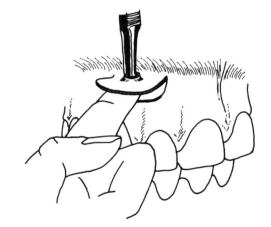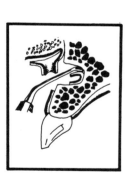

Fig. 98   This tube is closed with a mattress suture and the flap is replaced and sutured.

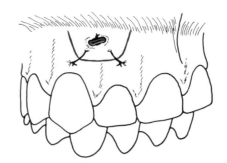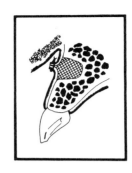

Fig. 99   **Removal of mucoceles**

These socalled cysts are most often found in the labial mucosa and in the floor of the mouth, where they may reach a considerable size. Only the small cysts in the labial and buccal mucosa are dealt with in this text. The treatment is surgical removal, but recurrence may be expected as a result of damage to and obstruction of adjacent salivary ducts. The operation starts with a semicircular incision along the base of the cyst.

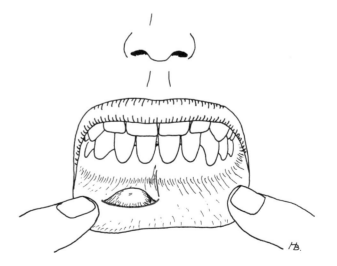

Fig. 100   By careful, blunt dissection the mucosa is detached from the cyst.

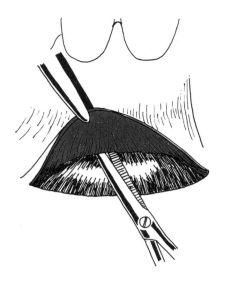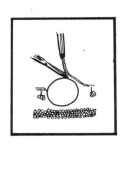

Fig. 101   When this dissection has been completed, the cyst including the associated minor salivary glands is disengaged using sharp dissection. As the cyst lining consists of only capsule of compressed connective tissue a perforation is often unavoidable. This will cause a collapse of the cyst which makes it difficult to remove. To help the dissection it may be advantageous to pack the cavity with gauze. The sutures are placed with an atraumatic needle in the mucosa only without interfering with the underlying salivary glands.

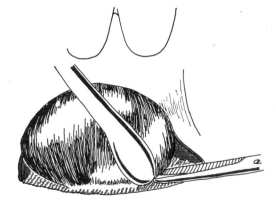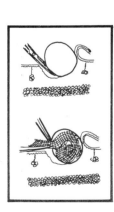

Fig. 102 Small and superficial mucoceles are removed by simple excision. An elliptical incision round the cyst facilitates a complete removal.

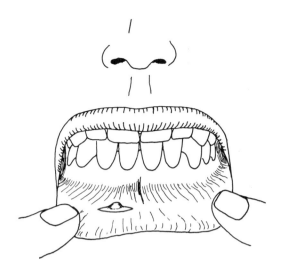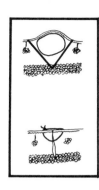

Exposure of impacted teeth

Impacted and semi-impacted teeth may somtimes be retained and brought into a normal functioning position in the dental arch by surgical exposure combined, if necessary, with orthodontic treatment. The need for such treatment is most relevant for the maxillary cuspid which is chosen as an example in the following text.

Fig. 103   The method of the operation is dependent on the position of the crown in relation to the oral mucosa. If the crown is easy to locate, an area of superjacent mucosa slightly larger than the extent of the crown is excised.

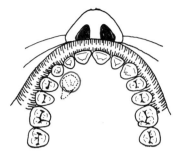

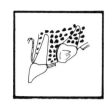

Fig. 104   Using a bur, the periphery of the crown is exposed and it is especially important that the cusp is uncovered. These superficially positioned canines may often erupt spontaneously after denudation. If active traction is necessary, this may be established as shown in Figs. 107–108. The wound is covered with a periodontal pack which may be removed in 14 days. The pack should be pressed well up round the periphery of the crown to prevent granulation tissue from the wound margins covering the opening.

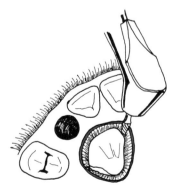

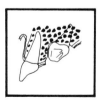

Fig. 105   If the cuspid is situated deep in the bone it may be difficult to determine where the opening in the mucosa should be placed. For this reason and to facilitate an adequate bone removal the palatal mucosa should be reflected after having made a marginal incision as shown in the drawing.

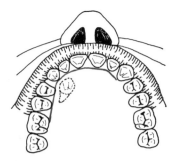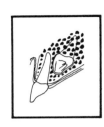

Fig. 106   A liberal amount of bone superjacent to the crown is removed along with the primary cuspid. It is important again to expose the cusp if this can be done without damaging the adjoining teeth. If the crown is situated close to the alvelous of the primary cuspid, this may be included in the cavity.

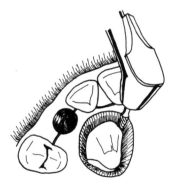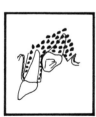

Fig. 107   As it is usually necessary to apply orthodontic traction on the tooth a point of fixation is mandatory. This may be done in several ways. One is to cement a stainless steel crown with a welded eye for attachment of an orthodontic ligature. The crown is fitted according to the usual principles. The correct size is determined by direct measuring on the exposed tooth. If the crown is easily accessible an orthodontic band may be used instead. The cementation is carried out using Ames red coppercement or a similar brand.

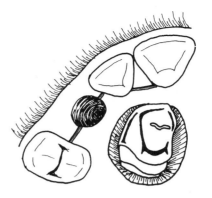

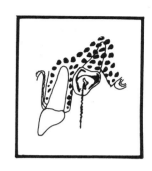

Fig. 108   Another possibility is to place a ligature of 0.4 mm stainless steel wire round the neck of the tooth. It is often difficult to pass the wire over the buccal surface, especially if the cusp is situated close to the roots of the incisors.

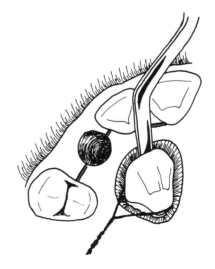

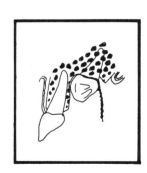

Fig. 109 The palatal mucosa is replaced and an opening is cut out corresponding to the size of the bone cavity. This may even include part of the marginal gingiva. The palatal flap is sutured and the exposed tooth is covered with a periodontal pack as described earlier (Fig. 104).

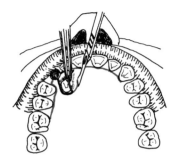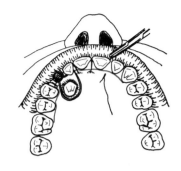

Fig. 110 The labially placed cuspid is often situated immediately deep to the oral mucosa and may therefore be exposed directly by cutting out an opening as shown on the figure. Note that the incision includes part of the labial fold.

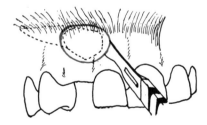

Fig. 111   The crown is exposed with a bur as previously described (Fig. 104).

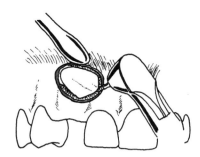

Fig. 112   The unattached mucosa in the labial fold must be secured with a mattress suture through the periosteum, otherwise the wound edge will tend to slide down and cover the exposed crown. Orthodontic traction is often necessary and a point of fixation is established as shown earlier in the text (Figs. 107–108). Finally a protective cover of periodontal pack is placed.

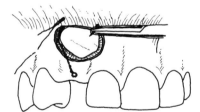

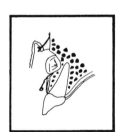

Fig. 113 The semi-impacted third mandibular molar may occasionally be brought to eruption by removing the distal soft tissue flap. It is a prerequisite however, that normal gingival conditions can be created all round the tooth. The operation is easy; the mucosal flap is simply cut off with a knife as shown on the drawing, and the wound is covered with a periodontal pack.

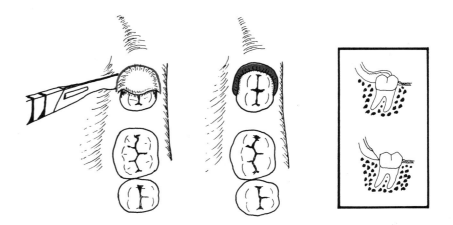

Removal of impacted teeth

These operations are difficult to describe in complete detail in view of the many variations in position and root anatomy. The following examples are therefore only intended to supply guidelines for choosing the right method of operation in each individual case. Two important conditions for achieving a good result are 1) a careful planning of the operation based on a thorough clinical and radiologic examination and 2) to secure a free line of extraction before commencing the removal of the tooth. There should be minimal bone removal and it is often less traumatic to divide the tooth in order to gain a free line of extraction for each part. The operation consists of the following phases:

1) Reflection of muco-periosteal flap
2) Exposure of the free line of extraction
3) Removal of tooth
4) Wound debridement and suture

Fig. 114 **The mandibular third molar**

Anatomical considerations. This tooth may be positioned in several different ways and the operative technique must therefore be adapted accordingly. Judged from the occlusal plane, 5 main positions can be found. These are the vertical, mesio-angular, disto-angular, horizontal and atypical positions. As far as the last group is concerned the operations may be very difficult and to such an extent that a description is outside the scope of the present manual. Only the four first-mentioned categories will be dealt with. The anatomical structures relevant for these operations are mentioned in the drawing. Note the line of incision from the anterior border of the ramus. The cut is made through the buccinator muscle and part of the tendon of the temporalis muscle. It is important that the incision is not placed too far medially, where the retromolar artery in the retromolar fossa or even worse, the lingual nerve, may be cut. The lingual nerve is situated close to the lingual bone in the third molar area and is also liable to be damaged later in the operation. Finally it should be mentioned that the inferior alveolar nerve often runs in close relation to the roots of the third molar, in rare cases even penetrating these.

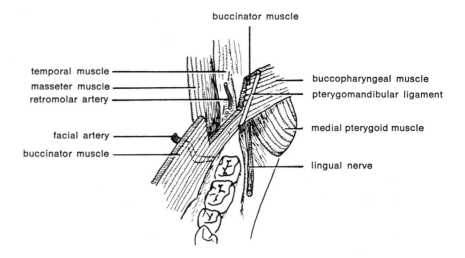

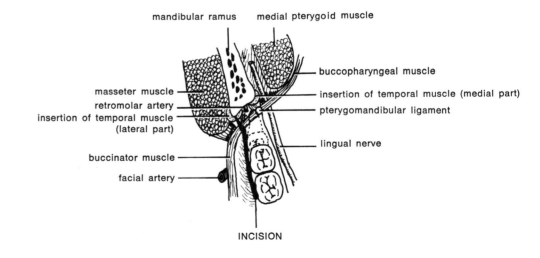

74

Fig. 115   The line of incision is similar in the four categories. It starts at the anterior border of the ramus and continues as a marginal incision buccal to the second and the first molars. On rare occasions when dealing with extremely deep retentions it may be necessary to apply an angular line of incision in order to get a good view of the operative field. The vertical incision is placed at the mesial end of the marginal incision. Reflection of the muco-periosteal flap is started in the region of the first molar and continued distally to the anterior border of the ramus, where it may be found necessary to divide the tendon of the temporalis muscle with a pair of scissors to get an adequate bone exposure.

Fig. 116   The lingual flap is often adherent to the dental sac and must be dissected. The field of operation is exposed as shown on the right side of the figure. The periosteal elevator in this position protects the lingual nerve during operation.

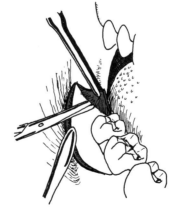
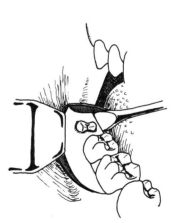

Fig. 117 *The vertical position.* Vertically situated third molars with a normal root anatomy as shown on the drawing can often be removed without too much difficulty as the free line of extraction may be secured by bone removal alone. The muco-periosteal flaps buccally and lingually are reflected as shown in the two preceding drawings.

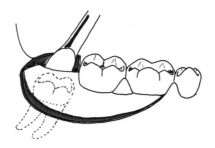

Fig. 118 The bone cover is removed in such a way that the prominence of the tooth is exposed. To secure a free line of extraction it is especially important to remove an adequate amount of bone distal to the crown because the distally curved roots force the tooth to be removed in that direction.

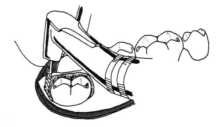

Fig. 119   When the crown is adequately exposed, a straight elevator is placed mesially as close to the neck of the tooth as possible. With cautious rotating movements of the elevator the tooth is lifted out of the socket. If after the initial loosening the tooth encounters the distal bone, the elevator may be placed buccally to lift the tooth out in a lingual direction.

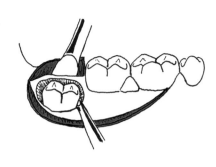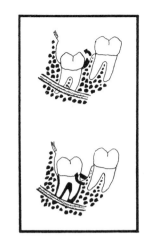

Fig. 120   If the roots of the vertically situated wisdom tooth are curved as shown on the drawing, the tooth must be divided and each root removed in the most favourable direction having regard to its curvature. The roots are separated applying a large bur which leaves the space necessary for adequate freedom of motion. The tilting of the bur must follow that of the crown to avoid perforation of the lingual bone.

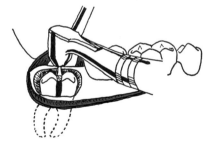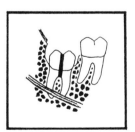

Fig. 121   In view of the comparatively limited motions possible when removing the first fragment it is advisable to start elevating the least curved root of the two – in this case the distal one. As shown on the right of the drawing, the removal takes place in two stages. First the root is luxated by moving the crown mesially, followed by a reversed rotation lifting the root out of the socket.

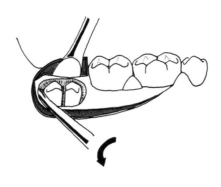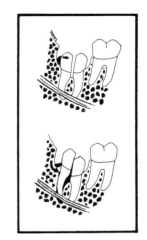

Fig. 122   The mesial fragment is removed in distal direction where adequate space has been created.

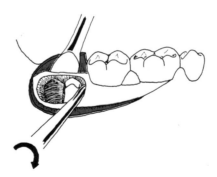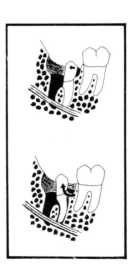

Fig. 123   All bony edges and areas where elevators have been supported should be smoothed with a file. The field of operation is irrigated with saline especially in the crevice between the buccal flap and the mandible where remnants of bone or tooth may hide. A tight suture is placed behind the second molar to keep the flap from sliding upwards. This suture should hold the mucosa beneath the prominence of the tooth. A second suture is placed on top of the cavity as a horizontal mattress suture.

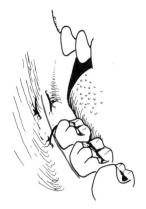

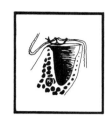

Fig. 124   *The mesio-angular position.* A tooth in this position has a more or less pronounced tilting of the crown in mesial direction. In this way the mesial cusps are locked against the distal surface of the second molar. This makes it impossible to clear the line of extraction by bone removal alone. The flap reflection is done in the usual manner.

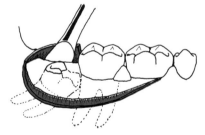

Fig. 125 After exposure of the crown the mesial part is split off with a bur and the fragment removed with an elevator.

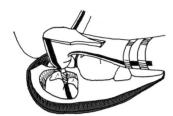 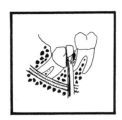

Fig. 126 With a straight or contra-angular elevator supported in the mesial part of the cavity the rest of the tooth is removed in distal direction. This line of extraction calls for an adequate enlargement of the pericoronal space in the distal part.

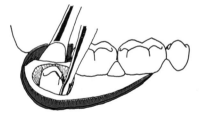 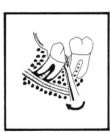

Fig. 127 Partition of the mesio-angular wisdom tooth is often easier and more rapidly done with a chisel. After the partition the distal part is removed first followed by the mesial fragment. Suturing is done as shown in Fig. 123.

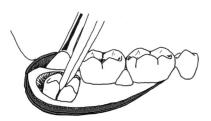

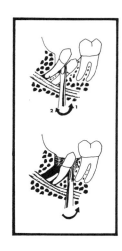

Fig. 128 *The disto-angular position.* This type can be more difficult to remove than the operator is led to believe by judging from the radiograph alone. The crown is locked in a bony cavity beneath the anterior border of the ramus while the root is situated close to the distal root of the second molar. The flap reflection is done in the usual manner.

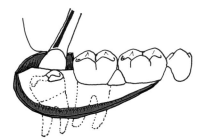

Fig. 129   In view of the afore-mentioned conditions it is impossible to remove the tooth intact unless there is a considerable amount of bone reduction. It is therefore less traumatic to cut off the distal part of the crown using bur or chisel and remove the fragment separately. This requires only a moderate bone resection.

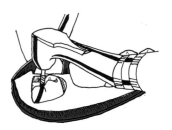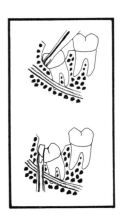

Fig. 130   The larger mesial part of the tooth may now be removed by elevation from the mesial side. In spite of this partition the crown may often engage the distal wall of bone during the last stage of elevation. In these cases the elevator is shifted to the buccal side and the tooth is guided out of the socket in lingual direction thereby avoiding the distal overhang of bone.

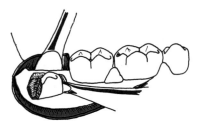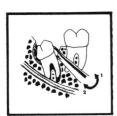

Fig. 131   If the tooth shows a pronounced disto-angular tilt or is deeply embed-
ded in bone, it is better to cut off the entire crown and remove it. In
this way more space is created for elevating the rest of the tooth.

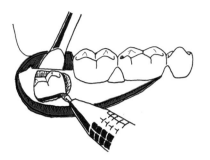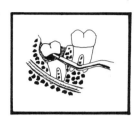

Fig. 132   Using a bur, part of the mesio-buccal bone is removed to make room
for a point of elevation in the root surface. With a contraangled
elevator placed herein the rest of the tooth is elevated in distal direction.
If the roots are diverging grossly from the line of extraction, it may be
necessary to section and remove them one at a time.

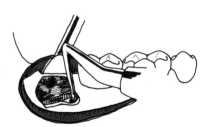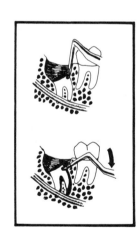

Fig. 133   *The horizontal position.* The horizontally impacted wisdom tooth is almost always placed with the crown in close relation to the distal surface of the second molar. The flap reflection is done in the usual manner.

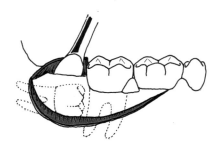

Fig. 134   After exposing the superficial part of the crown the tooth is partitioned with a large fissure bur at the cemento-enamel junction. In order to be able to remove the coronal part, this fragment should be wider at the top than at the bottom and the cut should therefore be made with a distal inclination.

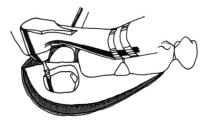 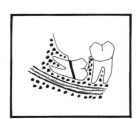

Fig. 135   As the mandibular canal is often situated in close relation to the tooth the cut is not carried through completely. The last bridge of dentin is fractured with a Barry's elevator as shown in the drawing.

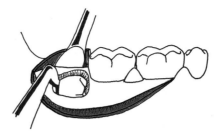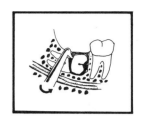

Fig. 136   The crown is pushed distally as far as the width of the cut permits. The cusps are thereby disengaged and the crown may be lifted out of the cavity.

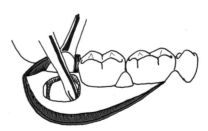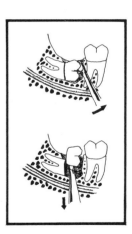

Fig. 137   A hole is drilled into the distal root. Barry's elevator is placed in it and with the distal bone as support the roots are pulled forward in the cavity from where they are turned and removed.

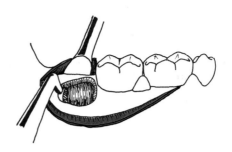
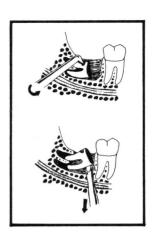

Fig. 138   **The maxillary third molar**
The greatest difficulty in removing this wisdom tooth is the inadequate survey of the region. The technical problems are seldom of any special magnitude when due consideration is given to the close relation to the maxillary sinus and to the cancellous bone which prohibits any excessive force being applied. The tooth is usually situated in a slightly mesio-angular position with the occlusal surface pointing in buccal direction. The same technique may therefore be applied in most cases.

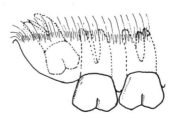
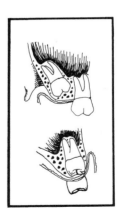

Fig. 139　An angular incision is used which is started off in the pterygomaxillary sulcus and carried forward to the mesial aspect of the second molar from where the vertical incision is extended.

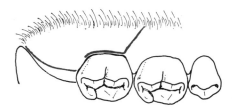

Fig. 140　The buccal muco-periosteal flap is reflected and a bur is used to expose the crown round both the occlusal and the buccal surfaces. It is sometimes necessary to reflect the palatal mucosa too, in order to expose the occlusal surface properly.

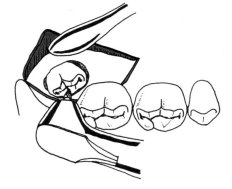

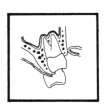

Fig. 141 Using a straight or contra-angled elevator from the mesial side the tooth is removed in buccal direction, possibly with a slight distal rotation during the last phase. The elevator is supported by the buccal bone and the disto-buccal root of the second molar. This support is weak and only a limited force may be applied. If the tooth is firmly fixed, the crown should be uncovered completely and the extraction performed with forceps.

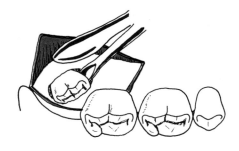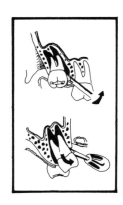

Fig. 142 The sutures are placed as shown in the figure. It is important to secure the corner of the flap primarily to achieve a correct replacement of the flap.

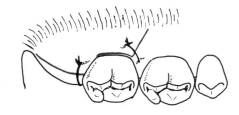

Fig. 143 **The maxillary cuspid**

The palatal position is by far the most frequent one and often gives rise to operative difficulties. This position is therefore chosen as an example for the description of the operation. If the cuspid is situated buccally, it may be removed according to the guidelines for the mandibular cuspid (Figs. 149–153) with the exception that a U-shaped incision at an adequate distance from the crown is used instead.

The removal of the palatally positioned cuspid is started off with a marginal incision from the first molar on the same side to the cuspid on the other side. The palatal muco-periosteal flap is reflected cutting the neurovascular bundle in the incisive foramen. This may be done without complications as the sensitivity in the area is eventually restored. The flap may conveniently be attached to one of the opposite molars as shown on the drawing.

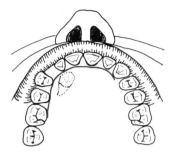
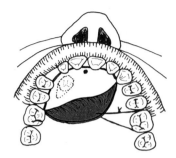

Fig. 144 The crown is exposed with bur to the largest possible extent. The line of extraction may now be open and the tooth can be elevated directly.

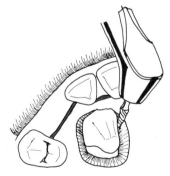
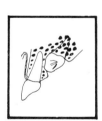

Fig. 145   If the crown is situated close to the roots of the incisors, the cusp may be impossible to expose without damaging the periodontia of these teeth. With a blocked line of extraction it is now necessary to partition the tooth at the cemento-enamel junction.

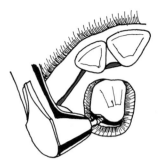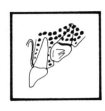

Fig. 146   To avoid damage to the periodontal structures of the incisors the cut is not carried all the way through the hard tissues, and the last bridge of dentin is fractured with the elevator. The crown may now be pushed in apical direction, whereby the cusp is disengaged from the bone. During removal of the crown the alveolar process should be supported with a finger in order to feel if too much force is being applied.

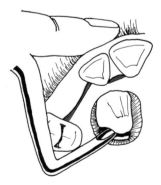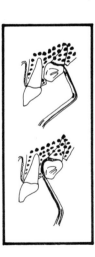

Fig. 147 A hole is drilled in the root surface for elevator engagement. Using the bone as support, the root can be extracted as shown to the right. If the root tip is curved or hypercementotic more bone must be removed to allow the freedom of motion necessary for extraction.

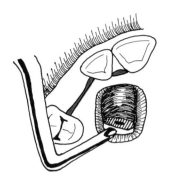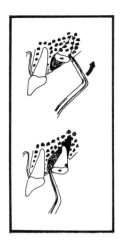

Fig. 148 The sutures are placed interdentally as shown. To avoid a subperiosteal formation of hematoma the palatal mucosa may be kept in place by a constructed acrylic plate.

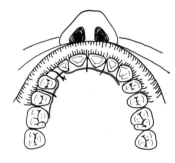

Fig. 149 **The mandibular cuspid**

The mandibular cuspid is most frequently retained in a labial position. In this situation it is mostly the horizontally or the obliquely placed cuspid which require surgical treatment. The horizontal impaction is chosen as an example in the following illustrations. – The operation begins with an angular incision.

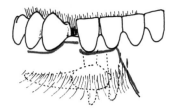

Fig. 150 After reflection of a muco-periosteal flap the crown is exposed. In most cases the crown can now be elevated directly.

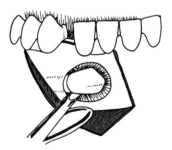

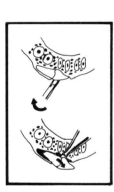

Fig. 151   If the line of extraction is blocked, for instance because of close relationship with the roots of the incisors, a partial division of the tooth
is done at the cemento-enamel junction, after which the crown is
fractured and removed.

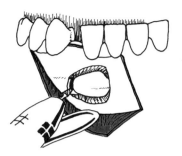
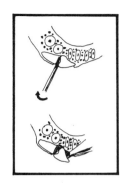

Fig. 152   The root is pulled forward into the bone cavity, turned outward and
removed.

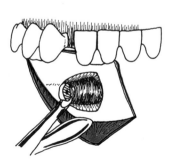
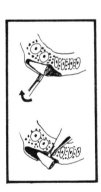

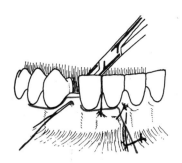

Fig. 153   The sutures are placed in the manner shown on the drawing. Note the usage of a straight needle for the interdental sutures.

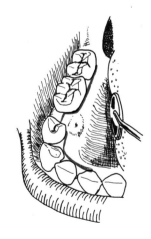

Fig. 154   **The second mandibular premolar**
This tooth is most frequently retained in a vertical position lingual to the dental arch, where the crown may be directly palpated. A marginal incision is adequate for exposing the field of operation because of the concavity of the mandibular body. The length of the incision may be seen from the drawing.

Fig. 155　The reflection of the muco-periosteal flap must be done very cautiously as the mucosa is thin and easily torn. The crown is exposed with due consideration to the marginal bone of the adjacent teeth.

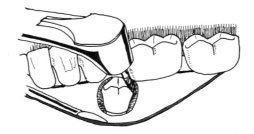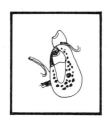

Fig. 156　In view of the wedging between the adjacent teeth it is often impossible to achieve a free line of extraction without partitioning, which is done at the neck of the tooth as indicated.

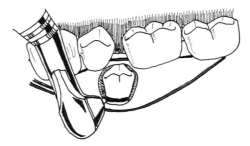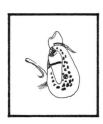

Fig. 157 The bridge of dentin which is left buccally is fractured and the crown removed with an elevator.

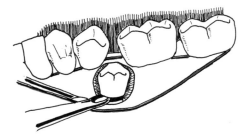
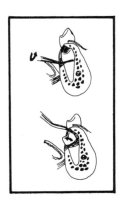

Fig. 158 The root is elevated and removed in a lingual direction. If it is firmly fixed a point of purchase is drilled into the exposed surface mesially, and the root may now be lifted up using the bone shelf as support for a contra- angled elevator.

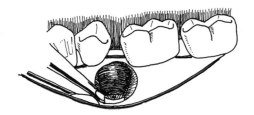
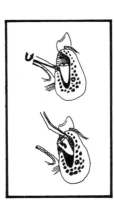

Fig. 159   The incision is closed with interdental sutures placed with a straight needle.

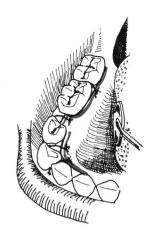

Fig. 160   **The supernumerary tooth**

Supernumerary teeth are most frequently found in the midline of the maxilla palatally to the permanent incisors. Their position may vary a great deal and they are often inverted. They may cause retention of one or both permanent central incisors. The removal should therefore be carried out during the normal eruption period of these teeth. In many cases, however, the supernumerary tooth or teeth may not be discovered until later when failing eruption of one or both permanent incisors leads to a radiologic examination.

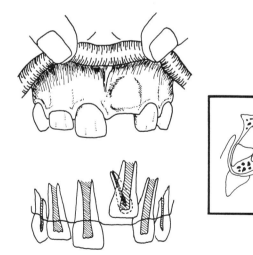

Fig. 161 As the supernumerary tooth is often located deeply in the bone close to the floor of the nasal cavity, problems may arise in achieving adequate local analgesia, as the bone in this area is partly innervated by ramifications from the nasopalatine nerve. These ramifications branch off in the incisive canal and are therefore not influenced by the normal deposition of analgesic solution in the incisive foramen. This may therefore be supplemented with an injection into the canal itself. The needle is advanced into the canal, where a small deposit is placed in the upper part. If it is difficult to locate the canal, the analgesia may be performed after reflection of the soft tissue when the opening is clearly visible. Another possibility is to place a cotton applicator moistened with a topical analgesic on both sides of the nasal septum, where the nasopalatine nerve is situated immediately deep to the thin mucosal lining.

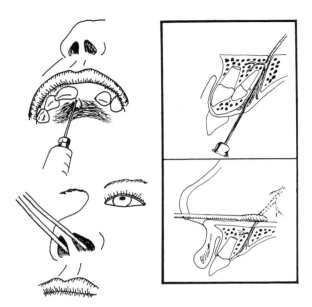

Fig. 162 The operation is started off with a marginal incision palatally as indicated in the figure.

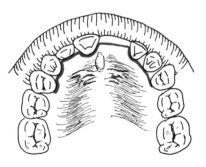

Fig. 163 The muco-periosteal flap is reflected and the crown and the neck of the supernumerary tooth are exposed. This must be done carefully so as not to damage the permanent tooth especially in the apical area. If the supernumerary tooth is small and situated in a normal position, it may be removed with an elevator. If the tooth is inverted or wedged between the incisors, partitioning is done at the cemento-enamel junction as shown in the example of the impacted cuspid (Figs. 145–146), and the tooth is removed in two pieces.

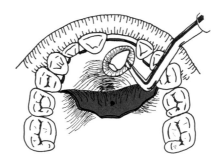 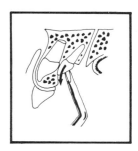

Fig. 164 Sutures are placed interdentally. In most cases of a simultaneous impaction of the permanent central incisor, exposure of the crown of this tooth is indicated. This is done according to the same guidelines as for the labially impacted cuspid (Fig. 110–112). It is, however, seldom that orthodontic traction is necessary.

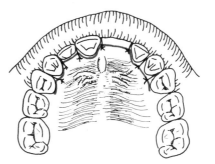 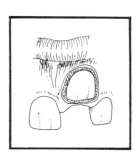

Transplantation of teeth

Transplantation of teeth from one site to another in the same individual (auto-transplantation) is now based on well documented scientific principles which makes it reasonable to recommend its use more widely. Certain requirements must, however, be adhered to. The transplant should have a wide open apical foramen with approximately 2/3 of the root having being formed. Furthermore all other possibilities for treatment (orthodontic, endodontic or prosthetic) should be evaluated.

The treatment consists of the following phases:

1) Preparation of recipient site
2) Removal of donor tooth
3) Moving the transplant to recipient site
4) Fixation of the transplant
5) Extended follow-up of the transplant

Fig. 165   As an example we have chosen a transplantation of the mandibular third molar to the first molar socket. This treatment may be indicated relatively often because of the high incidence of extensive caries in the first molar, but transplantation of premolars may also be indicated in cases of aplasia. The drawing shows a situation where there are reasonable indications for transplantation. It is important to measure the space available on the radiograph to be sure that the mesio-distal width of the transplant does not exceed that of the tooth to be extracted.

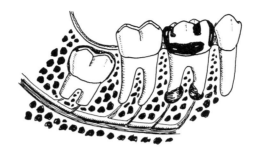

Fig. 166   The operation starts with the type of incision used for removal of impacted wisdom teeth with the modification that the interdental papillae are included in the buccal flap. The gingiva lingual to the first molar is gently reflected to avoid trauma during the extraction which is carried out with great caution.

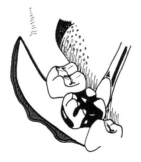

Fig. 167 The interradicular septum is removed to secure adequate space for the transplant. Where periapical granulomas or cysts are present these are curetted and the socket is covered with gauze to prevent accumulation of saliva.

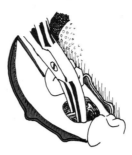 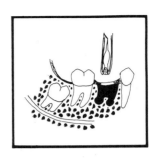

Fig. 168 The third molar is exposed to a larger extent than usual, so that the removal may take place without damage. The tooth is gently loosened with an elevator and lifted out of the socket with a forceps.

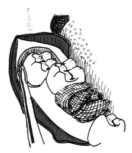 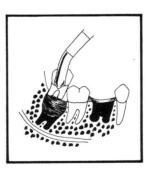

Fig. 169 The transplant is placed immediately in the empty socket of the first molar. The roots should be clear of the alveolar bone in order to avoid damage to the epithelial sheath of Hertwig. If further bone removal is necessary the transplant should be kept in sterile saline during that procedure. Note that the tooth is placed in slight infraocclusion. The gingiva is sutured tightly round the tooth.

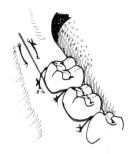 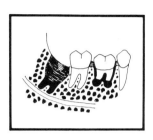

Fig. 170 Two orthodontic bands connected with a 0.9 mm soft stainless steel wire buccally and lingually are cemented on the adjacent teeth. This apparatus of fixation is made preoperatively. The wires are bent into contact with the tooth to which the apparatus is secured using cold curing acrylic. This acrylic bandage must not come into occlusion nor contact the marginal gingiva. A strict regime of oral hygiene is important to avoid periodontal complications. The fixation can be removed after 4 weeks. The transplant should be followed clinically and radiologically at regular intervals of 1–2 months.

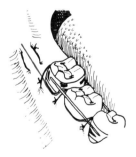 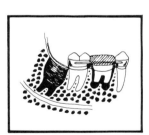

Extirpation of labial and lingual frena

It is often necessary to eliminate labial or lingual frena for orthodontic, prosthetic or periodontal reasons.It is when the frenum is inserted close to the crest of the alveolar process or in the marginal gingiva, causing adverse pull on the oral mucosa, that surgical treatment is indicated.

Fig. 171 Extirpation of the labial frenum is started off with two parallel incisions from its attachment to the upper lip to the incisive papilla. In the attached gingiva the incision is carried through to the bone while in the loosely attached part only the submucosa and muscular tissues are involved.

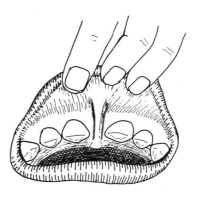

Fig. 172 Using a periosteal elevator or curette the labial frenum is disengaged in its full length between the labial mucosa and the palate.

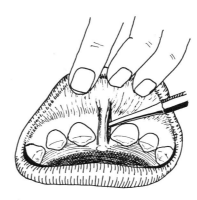

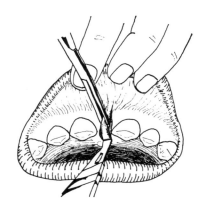

Fig. 173   The frenum is grasped with a hemostat, lifted outward and cut anterior to the incisive papilla.

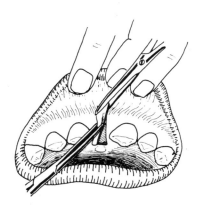

Fig. 174   The final cut is made with a pair of scissors in the labial sulcus and the frenum is removed completely.

Fig. 175　A single suture is placed in the mobile part of the wound edges. The suture should engage the periosteum to secure the depth of the sulcus. A gauze compress is placed between the incisors to obtain hemostasis. This compress may be removed shortly after the operation. A periodontal pack is usually not necessary as the bone is quickly covered by granulation tissue.

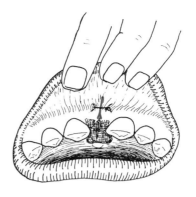

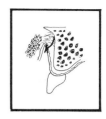

Fig. 176　Surgical correction of the lingual frenum is a minor operation. As shown in the drawing, however, the frenum is located close to the deep lingual vein and the submandibular duct which may be damaged by careless operative technique.

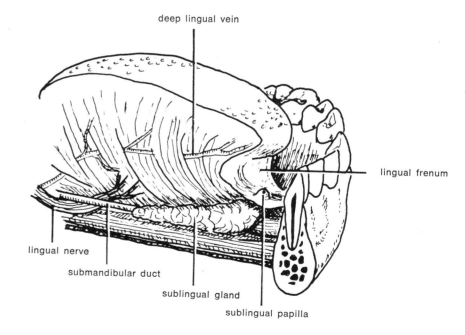

deep lingual vein

lingual frenum

lingual nerve

submandibular duct

sublingual gland

sublingual papilla

Fig. 177 The tongue is pulled forward and upward cutting the tight lingual frenum at the base of the tongue with a pair of scissors.

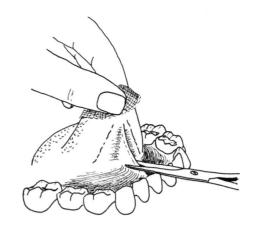

Fig. 178 The resulting rhomboid defect is closed with interrupted sutures starting at the base of the tongue. As the oral mucosa is very thin in that location, an atraumatic suture is preferable.

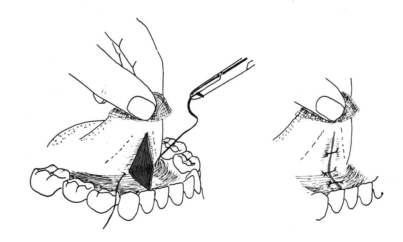

Preprosthetic surgery

The primary shaping of the alveolar process after extraction of teeth is a prerequisite for creating optimal conditions for a possible prosthetic treatment. Secondary alterations, which may have been caused by unstable or otherwise inappropriate dentures, must also be corrected. Those procedures described in this manual are only minor preprosthetic operations, as larger vestibuloplasties, bone transplantations and so on are rarely done in general practice.

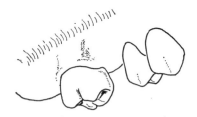

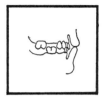

Fig. 179 Alveolar ridge contouring

Sometimes the alveolar bone around isolated teeth projects above the adjacent parts of the alveolar ridge or may show a heavy, especially buccally directed, prominence. After extraction of such teeth it is therefore necessary to make a correction of the remaining collar of bone to ensure a smooth base for the denture.

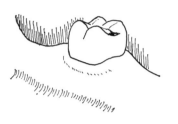

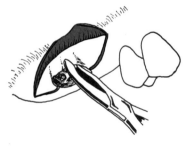

Fig. 180 In the mandible a 1 cm long incision is made mesially and distally to the socket and lingual and buccal flaps are reflected. In the maxilla, where the buccal alveolar plates project more extensively, it may be necessary to use an angular incision in order to expose the bone sufficiently to do an adequate reduction. The palatal bone seldom requires correction and for this reason only the buccal flap needs to be reflected. The projecting edges of bone are removed with a *rongeur,* and the area is smoothed with a file.

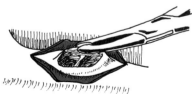

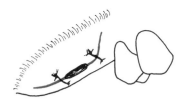

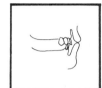

Fig. 181 The gingival margins are trimmed with a pair of scissors so that a complete adaptation in relation to the reduced foundation of bone is reached. The sutures are placed mesial and distal to the socket without attempting to obtain a complete closure over that cavity.

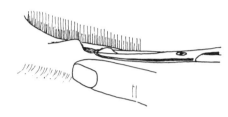

Fig. 182 Following multiple extractions a correction of the alveolar ridge is often required to obtain a good denture base. This modelling includes contouring of bone spicules, elimination of absolute undercuts and levelling of the alveolar process. These procedures are mandatory in cases where marginal periodontitis has caused bone resorption resulting in an irregular alveolar process.

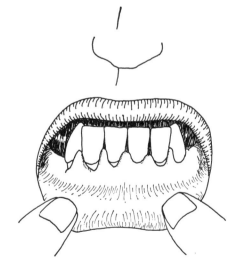

Fig. 183　Following the extractions all the papillae are sectioned along the crest of the alveolar process and the cut is carried 1 cm further backward on each side. The marginal mucosa is reflected taking care not to extend to the unattached gingiva, lest there be a reduction of the sulcus depth.

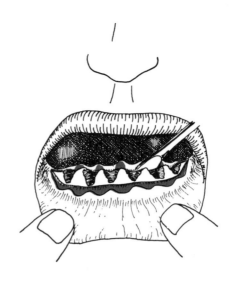

Fig. 184　The larger spicules and irregularities are removed using a *rongeur*. Care must be exercised to preserve as much bone as possible and an actual reduction in height must be avoided. The beaks of the *rongeur* must therefore be kept parallel to the bone surface as shown on the drawing.

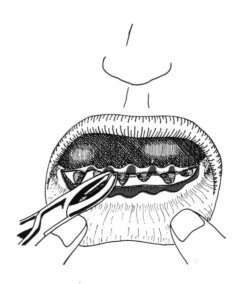

Fig. 185 Using a bone file the final contouring is done, the result of which may be assessed by palpation.

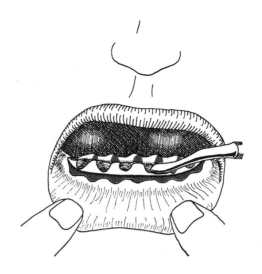

Fig. 186 The gingival margins and larger accumulations of granulation tissue are trimmed with a pair of scissors, so that the papillae may be adapted evenly over the interdental septa.

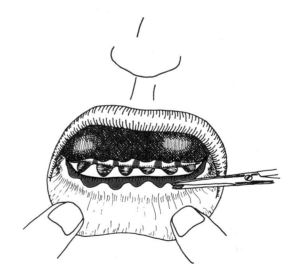

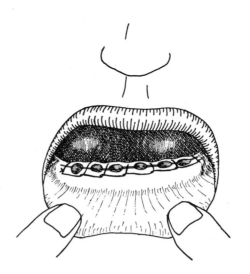

Fig. 187　The interdental papillae are replaced and sutured using a continuo us suture. This must not be tightened, as it is not intended to cover the openings of the alveoli. The method described here may also be used when inserting an immediate denture.

Fig. 188　**Intraalveolar resection**
In connection with insertion of immediate dentures a simpler method of bone reduction may be used in the maxilla. It is often a problem that the labial flange of the denture tends to stretch the upper lip and thereby change the appearance of the patient. This esthetic problem can be solved, without sacrificing any bone, in the following way. After extraction of the teeth all the tips of the interdental papillae are removed.

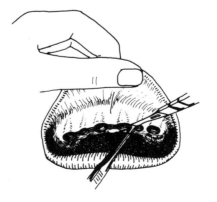

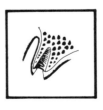

Fig. 189 Using a bone bur all interdental septae are removed. It is important that the removal is extended all the way to the depths of the sockets. In the most distally placed sockets a bone cut is made through the labial cortical plate. During this procedure the labial mucosa is covered with a finger in order to feel when the bur penetrates the bone so as to stop before any damage is done to the soft tissue. If an edentulous area is present, where atrophy of the alveolar process has already occurred, the intraalveolar resection is carried out as shown on the drawing in the lower right corner.

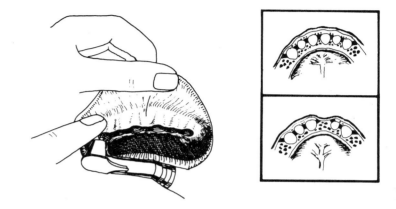

Fig. 190 Finally the resected part of the alveolar process is grasped with the fingers of both hands and pressure exerted on the labial plate which is fractured along the base of the alveolus. The labial prominence is thereby reduced. Suturing is unneccessary and the immediate denture may, after any possible corrections, be inserted. The laboratory technician has, of course, made similar alterations in the labial area of the plaster model to get a close fit of the denture. It must be noted that this operation cannot be used if it is neccessary to remove some of the teeth operatively. The fractured bone plate depends for its blood supply upon the covering mucosa, and if this has been reflected during a flap operation the bone will become necrotic.

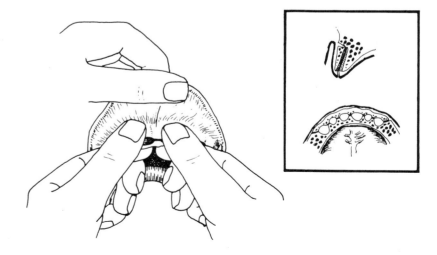

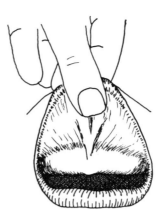

Fig. 191 Correction of labial and buccal frena
The resorption of the alveolar process, which is influenced by many factors, may progress to such an extent that labial and buccal frena come to insert close to the crest of the alveolar ridge and thereby exert an unfavourable influence on the retention of the denture. The mode of operation may depend on the shape of the frenum. In cases of thin, clearly outlined frena an extirpation is performed. A V-shaped incision is made according to the line of insertion on the alveolar process.

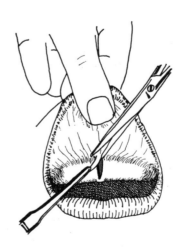
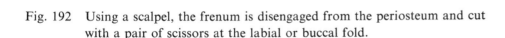

Fig. 192 Using a scalpel, the frenum is disengaged from the periosteum and cut with a pair of scissors at the labial or buccal fold.

Fig. 193 The resulting rhomboid wound is closed with interrupted sutures. To secure the depth of the sulcus the first suture is placed in the labial fold and penetrates the periosteum as well. The denture is corrected in the area using cold curing, soft acrylic or other temporary relining material, until the proper relining can be made usually after 3–4 weeks.

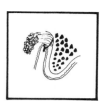

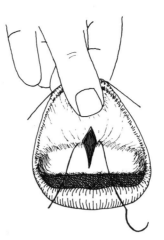

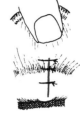

Fig. 194 A labial or buccal frenum with a broad base towards the sulcus is corrected using a localized vestibuloplasty. The operation is started off with a semicircular incision as shown in the figure.

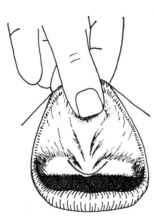

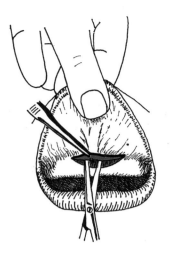

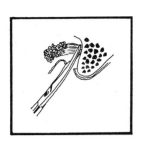

Fig. 195 Using a pair of scissors the frenum is dissected and disengaged from the periosteum cutting possible muscular attachments in the process.

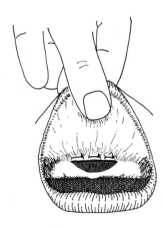

Fig. 196 The mobile wound edge is fastened in line with the adjacent parts of the labial sulcus using horizontal mattress sutures. An open wound is left for healing by second intention. The denture should preferably not be inserted during the period of healing, as a mechanical irritation of the wound may cause tissue hyperplasia. If the denture has to be worn, the margin should be relined as mentioned earlier (Fig. 193).

Fig. 197 Removal of fibrous hyperplasia

The fibrous hyperplasia of the mucosa on the alveolar process is most frequently seen in the molar region of he maxilla. In this location it may take up all of the intermaxillary space during occlusion or create absolute undercuts. Both conditions may seriously affect the construction of a removable denture. Before contemplating the reduction of hyperplastic tissue a radiograph should be taken to rule out the possibility of a retained third molar or an osseous overgrowth. In order to reduce the size of the fibrous tissue an elliptical incision is made from the pterygomaxillary fold as far mesially as the hyperplastic tissue indicates. The width of the incision depends on the extent of the fibrous hyperplasia; the greater the mass, the broader the incision, but caution is advisable as a final correction can be made just before the sutures are placed.

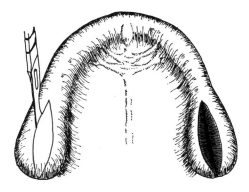 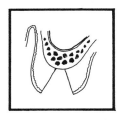

Fig. 198 The triangular piece of tissue is removed and the wound edges are undermined with a scalpel removing just enough tissue to obtain a normal thickness of the mucosa.

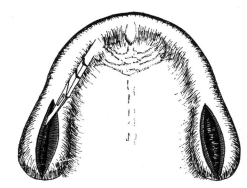 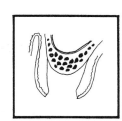

Fig. 199 The result is assessed by pressing the wound edges against each other and any possible surplus of tissue is removed with a pair of scissors. A continuous suture is placed. The denture is temporarily relined in that area with tissue conditioner.

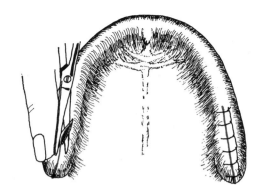 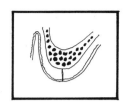

Fig. 200 Removal of denture hyperplasia

The soft tissue hyperplasia caused by ill-fitting dentures may occur in three different places. 1) on the crest of the alveolar ridge owing to resorbtion of underlying bone ("flabby ridge"), 2) in the buccal or labial fold owing to trauma from an overextended denture ("curtains") and 3) in the palate with a pebbly or granular texture resulting from irritation and Candida-infection ("denture stomatitis").

The fibrous, mobile alveolar ridge may be removed by making a narrow, elliptical incision along the excess soft tissue, which is grasped with a hemostat and disengaged from the periosteum.

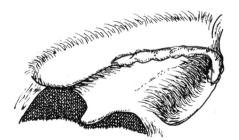 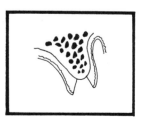

Fig. 201 The wound edges are adapted and possibly trimmed with a pair of scissors, cutting excess tissue as shown on the drawing. Occasionally a sharp, jagged alveolar ridge may be palpated. This can be exposed after incising and reflecting the periosteum and the bone edge smoothed with a file.

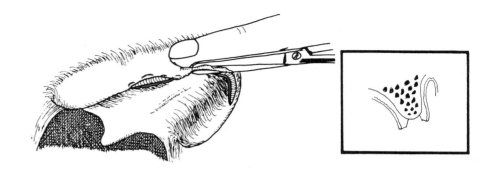

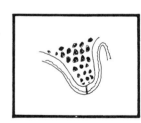

Fig. 202 A continuous suture is placed keeping the single turns close together for reasons of hemostasis in the briskly bleeding tissue. The denture should be relined with a tissue conditioner to avoid a recurrence.

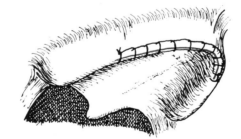

Fig. 203   In the mandible, where the hyperplasia is often ribbon-shaped, a simple cut using a pair of scissors is sufficient. Suturing is not necessary. Thin, well defined tissue hyperplasia in the labial or buccal fold may get the same treatment, while removal of larger accomulations of pathologic tissue in these regions must be combined with a vestibuloplasty to a sometimes considerable extent. Removal of palatal hyperplastic tissue is difficult and results in a large wound surface.

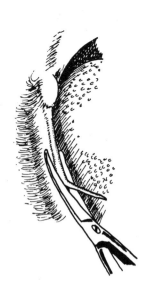

Closure of sinus perforation

Operations involving the maxillary sinus are normally outside the range of the general dental practitioner. An exception from this may be the closure of a sinus perforation created in connection with tooth extraction, where the operation constitutes a natural continuation of that treatment and where no previous pathological condition exists in the antrum calling for referral to a specialist. The treatment of a chronic oro-antral fistula or dislocated roots of teeth, which would involve the maxillary sinus itself in the procedure, should also be referred.

Fig. 204　As an example, a sinus perforation in the palatal alveolus of the first molar has been chosen. A buccal flap is used for the closure. A trapezoid incision is used which includes only the empty socket, but with the vertical incisions diverging towards the sulcus to ensure an optimal blood supply for the flap.

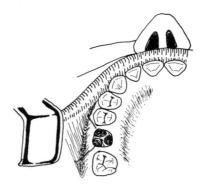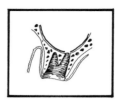

Fig. 205　The muco-periosteal flap must be reflected to such an extent, that the periosteum can be cut with a transverse incision beyond the buccal fold. This will increase the stretching capacity of the flap considerably.

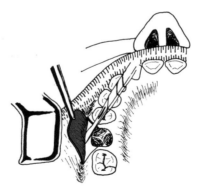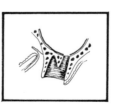

Fig. 206   To further ensure that the flap can be placed across the alveolus without any undue traction, a resection is carried out on the buccal plate. On the palatal side a partial reflection of the gingiva combined with removal of the pocket epithelium make sure that there will be adequate connective tissue contact between the flaps. The bone is finally smoothed with a file.

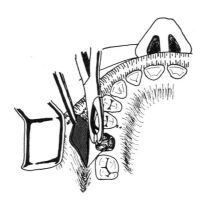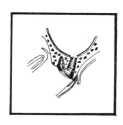

Fig. 207   Using horizontal mattress sutures the buccal and palatal wound edges are secured in close relation to each other while the remainder of the sutures are placed as normal interrupted sutures. The patient should be instructed not to blow his nose during the next 2 weeks and sneezing should be done with wide open mouth. Heavy suction during smoking should be prohibited.

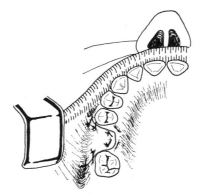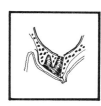

Biopsy

H. P. Philipsen

Biopsy is a simple procedure of considerable diagnostic value. The size, location and character of the lesion determines the type of procedure. Total excision or *excisional biopsy* including an adequate margin of normal tissue on all sides is preferable whenever the size of the lesion will permit its complete removal (Fig. 6). In this case biopsy is usually equivalent to treatment. When the lesion is too large to permit removal of the entire specimen, *incisional biopsy* is utilized. One or more representative sections are removed at the margin of the lesion including a portion of the adjacent normal tissue. Incisional biopsy procedures are demonstrated in the following illustrations.

Fig. 208 Colored antiseptics and topical analgetic agents should not be placed on the area to be removed. Avoid injecting analgetic solutions directly into the lesion as this procedure tends to distort the tissue. Block analgesia or infiltration around the periphery of the surgical site as shown should be used. Use of electrosurgical equipment that generates excessive heat usually results in distortion and is to be avoided.

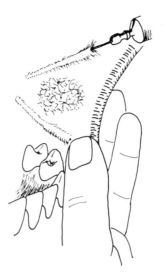

Fig. 209 The site of biopsy showing typical changes at a margin of the lesion is selected and elliptical, sharp scalpel incisions are made to include adjacent normal tissue, especially on the deep side of the lesion.

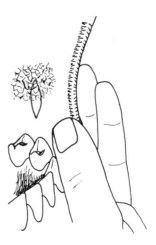
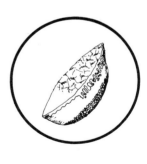

Fig. 210   The specimen is immobilized with tissue forceps and it should be grasped lightly in only one location to prevent crushing of the area to be studied microscopically. The specimen is dissected free with scissors or scalpel and the resulting wound is closed with interrupted sutures, to be removed 5 days postoperatively.

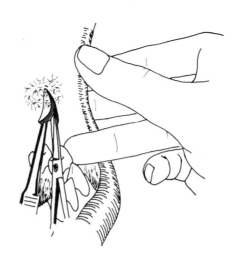

Fig. 211   Immediately after surgical removal, the specimen is placed in a large volume of fixative (10 per cent formalin, i.e. one part commercial formaldehyde to nine parts water). To avoid curling of the specimen during fixation mucous membrane biopsies are preferably stuck onto a piece of white cardboard using the fresh blood on the cut surface as glueing material.

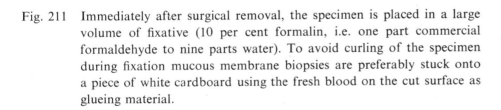

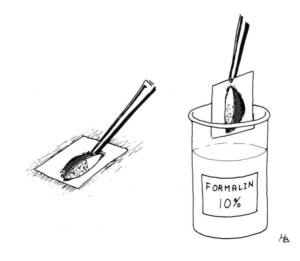

FORMALIN 10%

Fig. 212   In an intraosseous lesion, an incision is made through the mucoperiosteum and the flap is stripped away to expose the cortex. Lesional bone tissue is then removed using a trephine drill operating at low speed under sterile, saline irrigation. The bone cylinder is removed from the trephine drill using a dental probe and the specimen is immediately fixed as described previously.

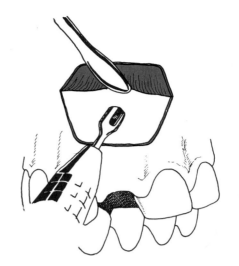
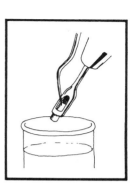

Index

Acrylic plate   91
Abscess, analgesia in   42
  chemotherapy in   42
  drainage of   44
  facially placed   44
  incision of   43
  lingually placed   46
  palatally placed   45
  treatment of   42
Alveolar ridge, contouring of   110
  after multiple extractions   111
  after single extractions   110
  by intraalveolar resection   114
Apicoectomy   47

Barry's elevator, application of 33,
  85, 86
Biopsy   126
  analgesia for   127
  excisional   10, 126
  incisional   127
Biopsy of bone   129
Bone file, application of   12
Bone, removal of   11
Bone spicules, removal of   127
Buccinator muscle   74
Bur, bone, application of   11
Bur, vulcanite, application of   51

Chemotherapy in treatment of
  abscess   42
Chisel, application of   11
  hand, application of   11
Curette, application of   49, 50, 51
Cuspid, mandibular, extraction of   30
  operative removal of   92

Cuspid, maxillary, exposure of   67
  extraction of   25
  operative removal of   89
Cyst, enuchleation of   54
  excision of   63
  extirpation of   54
  fenestration of   57
  marsupialization of   53
  surgical termination of   62
Cyst obturator, manufacturing of   59

Deep lingual veine   107
Denture, immediate, surgical
  treatment for   111, 114
  hyperplasia, excision of   120
  stomatitis, excision of   122
Denudation of tooth crown   66

Elevator, Barry, application of   33,
  85, 86
  contraangled, application of   36, 41,
  83, 90, 99,
  periosteal   11
  root pick, application of   26
  straight, application of   28, 38, 77,
  78, 80, 81, 82, 85, 88, 92, 93, 96
Endodontic surgery   47
Exposure, surgical, of tooth crown   66
Extirpation of labial frenum   105
  of lingual frenum   107
Extraction   23

Facial artery   74
Fibrous hyperplasia, excision of   119
Fistula, oro-antral   123

treatment of 48
Flap operation in the mandible 35
  in the maxilla 37
Flabby ridge, excision of 120
Forceps, cow horn 32
  lister 43
Forceps technique 23
Frenectomy 104

Gauze, hemostatic, application of 51
Greater palatine artery 45
Greater palatine nerve 45
Greater palatine veine 45

Handpiece, application of 11, 48, 50
  contraangled, miniature 51
Hemostat, application of 106

Impacted tooth, exposure of 66
  operative removal of 73
Incision 7
  angular 9
  elliptical 10, 127
  marginal 8, 75, 89
  suture of 12
  trapezoid 9
  U-formed 10
Incisive foramen 89, 98
Incisors, mandibular, extraction of 29
  maxillary, exposure of 99
  maxillary, extraction of 24
Intraalveolar septum, removal of 33,
  102

Kaplan instrument, application of 51
Knot, surgical 13

Labial and buccal frenae, correction
  of 116
  extirpation of 104
Lancet, application of 43
Lingual frenum, correction of 107
Lingual nerve 74
Luxation movements 23

Mallet, application of 11
Marsupialization of cyst 53
Mental foramen 35
Mucocele 63
Needle, curved 12
  straight 94
Needle holder, application of 13

Periodontal pack, application of 67
Preprosthetic surgery 109

Resection, intraalveolar 114
Retromolar artery 74
Rongeur, application of 11, 112
Root, operative removal of 34
  removal of 26, 27, 32
Root filling, retrograde 51
Root resection 47
Root tip, removal of 26
Root trunk, division of 27, 32
Rubberdam, application of 44

Scissors, application of 55, 75, 108,
  113, 116, 118, 122
Sinus perforation, closure of 123
Sublingual gland 107
Submandibular duct 107
Supernumerary tooth, analgesia for 98

removal of 98
Suture 12
  atraumatic 12
  continous 19
  interrupted 13
  mattress, horizontal 19
  mattress, vertical 18
  order of 18
  removal of 22
  material 12

Temporal muscle 74
Transplantation of teeth 100
Trephine drill, application of 129

Vertibuloplasty, local 117
Wisdom tooth, mandibular, extraction of
  31
  operative removal of 74
    vertical position 76
    mesio-angular position 79
    disto-angular position 81
    horizontal position 84
  transplantation of 101
Wisdom tooth, maxillary, extraction of
  29
  operative removal of 86
Wound debridement 12